Emergency Medicine: Avoiding the Pitfalls and Improving the Outcomes

This text is dedicated to the residents and faculty in Emergency Medicine at the University of Maryland Medical Center for providing the inspiration for this work; to my colleague Deepi Goyal, a true friend, scholar, and role model; to Mary Banks and Blackwell Publishing for supporting this work; to my children Nikhil, Eleena, and Kamran for providing the greatest inspiration in my life; and to my wife Sejal for her incredible support of all that I do, and without whom none of this would be possible.

Amal Mattu, MD

This text is dedicated to all those whose support and inspiration brighten my every day: to the Emergency Medicine residents, faculty, and nurses at Mayo Medical Center whose curiosity, patience, and passion benefits all those they touch; to Amal Mattu, a colleague, teacher, and mentor who I feel truly fortunate to call a friend; and most importantly to my wife Bhargavi and my children Kiran and Seeta whose unfailing support and understanding have made this all possible.

Deepi Goyal, MD

Emergency Medicine: Avoiding the Pitfalls and Improving the Outcomes

Edited by

Amal Mattu, MD
Program Director, Emergency Medicine Residency
Co-Program Director, Emergency Medicine/Internal
Medicine Combined Residency
Associate Professor of Emergency Medicine
University of Maryland School of Medicine
Baltimore, Maryland

and

Deepi Goyal, MD
Associate Program Director
Mayo Emergency Medicine Residency
Assistant Professor of Emergency Medicine
Mayo clinic College of Medicine
Rochester, Minnesota

4/08

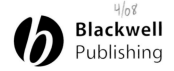
Blackwell Publishing

BMJ Books

Blackwell Publishing, Inc., 350 Main Street, Malden, Massachusetts
02148-5020, USA
Blackwell Publishing Ltd, 9600 Garsington Road, Oxford OX4 2DQ, UK
Blackwell Publishing Asia Pty Ltd, 550 Swanston Street, Carlton, Victoria 3053,
Australia

First published 2007
1   2007

Library of Congress Cataloging-in-Publication Data

Emergency medicine: avoiding the pitfalls and improving the outcomes/edited
by Amal Mattu and Deepi Goyal.
p.; cm.
Includes bibliographical references.
ISBN-13: 978-1-4051-4166-6 (pbk.:alk. paper)
1. Emergency medicine. I. Mattu, Amal. II. Goyal, Deepi.
[DNLM: 1. Emergencies. 2. Emergency Medicine. WB 105 E541 2007]
RC86.7.E4444 2007
616.02′5–dc22

                                    2006027486

ISBN: 978-1-4051-4166-6

A catalogue record for this title is available from the British Library

Set in 9/12 pt Meridien Roman by Charon Tec Ltd (A Macmillan Company),
Chennai, India
www.charontec.com
Printed and bound in Singapore by Markono Print Media Pte Ltd

Commissioning Editor: Mary Banks
Editorial Assistant: Victoria Pittman
Development Editor: Lauren Brindley
Production Controller: Rachel Edwards

For further information on Blackwell Publishing, visit our website:
http://www.blackwellpublishing.com

The publisher's policy is to use permanent paper from mills that operate a
sustainable forestry policy, and which has been manufactured from pulp
processed using acid-free and elementary chlorine-free practices. Furthermore,
the publisher ensures that the text paper and cover board used have met
acceptable environmental accreditation standards.

Blackwell Publishing makes no representation, express or implied, that the drug
dosages in this book are correct. Readers must therefore always check that any
product mentioned in this publication is used in accordance with the prescribing
information prepared by the manufacturers. The author and the publishers do
not accept responsibility or legal liability for any errors in the text or for the
misuse or misapplication of material in this book.

Contents

Contributors

Jeffrey Barrett, MD
Assistant Professor
Department of Emergency Medicine
Temple University School of Medicine
Philadelphia, PA

Joshua Broder, MD, FACEP
Associate Residency Program Director
Assistant Clinical Professor
Division of Emergency Medicine
Department of Surgery
Duke University Medical Center
Durham, NC

Michael A. DeAngelis, MD
Assistant Professor of Emergency Medicine
Department of Emergency Medicine
Temple University School of Medicine
Philadelphia, PA

Peter M. C. DeBlieux, MD
Professor of Clinical Medicine
Louisiana State University School of Medicine in
New Orleans
New Orleans, LA

Gus M. Garmel, MD, FACEP, FAAEM
Co-Program Director, Stanford/Kaiser EM Residency
Clinical Associate Professor
Emergency Medicine (Surgery)
Stanford University School of Medicine
and
Senior Emergency Physician
The Permanente Medical Group
Kaiser Santa Clara, CA

Richard A. Harrigan, MD
Associate Professor of Emergency Medicine
Department of Emergency Medicine
Temple University Hospital and School of Medicine
Philadelphia, PA

David J. Karras, MD, FACEP, FAAEM
Professor of Emergency Medicine
Associate Chair for Academic Affairs
Department of Emergency Medicine
Temple University School of Medicine
Philadelphia, PA

Anita L'Italien, MD
Chief Resident
Department of Emergency Medicine
University of North Carolina at Chapel Hill
Chapel Hill, NC

David E. Manthey, MD
Director, Undergraduate Medical Education
Associate Professor
Wake Forest University School of Medicine
Winston-Salem, NC

Joseph P. Martinez, MD
Assistant Professor of Emergency Medicine
Assistant Dean for Student Affairs
University of Maryland School of Medicine
Baltimore, MD

Siamak Moayedi, MD
Assistant Professor
Department of Emergency Medicine
University of Maryland School of Medicine
Baltimore, MD

Bret A. Nicks, MD
Assistant Medical Director
Wake Forest University School of Medicine
Winston-Salem, NC

Yesha Patel, MD
Assistant Professor, Emergency Medicine
Tufts University School of Medicine
Tufts-New England Medical Center
Boston, MA

Robert L. Rogers, MD, FAAEM, FACEP, FACP
Assistant Professor of Emergency Medicine
Director of Undergraduate Medical Education
The University of Maryland School of Medicine
Baltimore, MD

Jairo I. Santanilla, MD
Chief Resident
Louisiana State University School of Medicine in New Orleans
New Orleans, LA

Wayne A. Satz, MD
Associate Professor
Department of Emergency Medicine
Temple University
Philadelphia, PA

Stephen Schenkel, MD, MPP
Assistant Professor
University of Maryland School of Medicine
Baltimore, MD

Ghazala Sharieff, MD
Director of Pediatric Emergency Medicine
Palomar-Pomerado Health System/California Emergency
Physicians
and
Associate Clinical Professor
Children's Hospital and Health Center
University of California
San Diego, CA

Mercedes Torres, MD
Chief Resident
Department of Emergency Medicine
University of Maryland School of Medicine
Baltimore, MD

Kristine Thompson, MD
Clinical Instructor, Emergency Medicine
Department for Emergency Medicine
Mayo Clinic
Jacksonville, FL

Michael E. Winters, MD
Assistant Professor of Emergency Medicine and Medicine
Program Director, Combined Emergency Medicine/Internal
Medicine Training Program
University of Maryland School of Medicine
Baltimore, MD

Preface

Emergency Medicine is a high-risk specialty. The seasoned practitioner is well aware that that even the most mundane of patients may, at any moment, be on the brink of a catastrophic outcome. The emergency physician must, therefore, be ever wary of these "disasters in waiting." It seems that most pitfalls in emergency medicine, many of which result in medicolegal consequences, occur not purely due to a lack of knowledge but rather to simply "letting one's guard down."

This text was created in order to focus the attention of emergency physicians on these common pitfalls. The text is not comprehensive in scope, but rather it focuses the readers' attention on an assortment of chief complaints and patient groups that are frequently encountered in Emergency Medicine. The authors of each chapter were chosen for their expertise in the respective topics, and they have focused their text on potential pitfalls in everyday clinical practice that represent high risk for patient morbidity, mortality, and litigation. At the end of each chapter, they have provided important pearls for improving patient outcomes. Although the text is primarily intended for use by the seasoned practitioner, physicians-in-training should find many teaching points that will assist their education as well.

Finally, we hope that the reader will not relegate this text to the bookshelf alongside other voluminous, dusty reference books. Rather, we hope that the reader finds the text of appropriate size and practicality to read cover-to-cover and to use frequently during everyday practice in the Emergency Department and other acute-care settings.

Amal Mattu, MD
Deepi Goyal, MD

Chapter 1 | **Evaluation and Management of Patients with Chest Syndromes**

Richard A. Harrigan & Michael A. DeAngelis

Introduction

Chest pain is a common emergency department (ED) complaint with a well-known differential diagnosis. Yet compared to the abdomen, the chest contains relatively few structures (e.g., the heart, the lungs, the great vessels, the esophagus) to consider as the source of the complaint when evaluating a patient with chest pain. In these few structures, however, there exists the potential for several life-threatening maladies, some of which unfortunately occur rather commonly. In patients with chest pain, initial attention is often devoted to establishing the presence or absence of acute coronary syndrome (ACS), but indeed there are several other syndromes of critical importance and clinical relevance to consider. In this chapter, we consider six pitfalls related to ACS, followed by a variety of pitfalls related to other diseases of the chest: aortic dissection (AD), pulmonary embolism (PE), pericarditis, pneumothorax, esophageal rupture, and finally, herpes zoster.

Pitfall | **Over-reliance on the classic presence of chest pain for the diagnosis of acute myocardial infarction (MI)**

Although chest pain has long been considered the hallmark clinical feature of acute myocardial infarction (MI), it is important to recognize that the absence of chest pain in no way excludes the diagnosis. In a large observational study, Canto et al. examined the presenting complaints of nearly 435,000 patients with confirmed MI enrolled in the National Registry of Myocardial Infarction 2 (NRMI-2) database and found that one-third of the patients presented to the hospital without chest pain [1]. Other studies have reported similar findings. In one study, over 20% of 2096 patients diagnosed with acute MI presented with symptoms other than chest pain [2]. In another smaller study, nearly half (47%) of 721 patients hospitalized for acute MI presented to the ED without chest pain [3]. Risk factors associated with the absence of chest pain included age, female gender, non-white race, diabetes mellitus, and a prior history of congestive heart failure or stroke (see Table 1.1) [1].

| KEY FACT | **Over the age of 85, 60–70% of patients with acute MI present without chest pain.** |

Table 1.1 Risk factors for painless acute MI [1].

Risk Factors	% Without Chest Pain
Prior heart failure	51
Prior stroke	47
Age > 75 years	45
Diabetes mellitus	38
Non-white	34
Women	39

In the elderly population, chest pain is reported less frequently according to the NRMI-2 database, patients experiencing an acute MI without chest pain are, on average, 7 years older (74 versus 67 years) [1]. Uretsky et al. reported a mean age of 69.1 years in those patients without chest pain as compared to 58.7 years in those with chest pain [4]. Under the age of 85, chest pain is still present in the majority of patients but other non-pain symptoms (referred to as "anginal equivalents") such as shortness of breath, syncope, weakness, and confusion are common. Over the age of 85, 60–70% of patients with acute MI present without chest pain; shortness of breath is the most frequent anginal equivalent in this population [5].

Women are more likely than men to experience acute MI without chest pain [1–3, 6]. In one study, women over the age of 65 were the most prevalent group to experience acute MI without chest pain [6]. In another study of 515 women surveyed after experiencing an acute MI, only 57% reported chest pain at the time of their MI. The most frequent anginal equivalents reported were shortness of breath (58%), weakness (55%), unusual fatigue (43%), cold sweats (39%), and dizziness (39%) [7].

Patients with diabetes mellitus are at increased risk for acute MI and are more likely to present without chest pain [1, 8]. Medically unrecognized acute MI has been noted in up to 40% of patients with diabetes as compared to 25% of the non-diabetic population [8]. Although the NRMI-2 database noted that diabetics were more likely to experience acute MI without chest pain (32.6% versus 25.4%), two-thirds of those who experienced acute MI without chest pain were still non-diabetics [1].

Patients experiencing an acute MI without chest pain are more likely to suffer delays in their care. Analysis of the NRMI-2 database revealed that these patients were less likely to receive aspirin, heparin, or beta-adrenergic blockers in the initial 24 h and were much less likely to receive fibrinolysis or primary angioplasty (25.3% versus 74.0%) [1]. They were also more likely to die in the hospital compared to patients who presented with chest pain (23.3% versus 9.3%) [1]. Uretsky et al. reported a nearly 50% mortality rate in patients hospitalized with acute MI who presented without chest pain compared to an 18% mortality rate in those presenting with chest pain [4]. The 30- and 365-day mortality rates have also been noted to be higher in this group [2]. Clearly, populations other than diabetics are at risk to present without chest pain while having an acute MI; women and the elderly are among those groups identified to be at particular risk.

Pitfall | Exclusion of cardiac ischemia based on reproducible chest wall tenderness

ED visits for chest pain comprise 5–8% of all ED cases [9]. The etiologies of chest pain range from benign to life threatening. The goal of the emergency physicians (EP) is to identify the life-threatening causes, including acute MI. Ruling out acute MI in the clinically stable patient presenting with chest pain and a non-diagnostic ECG represents a particular challenge to the EP.

Certain chest pain characteristics have been shown to decrease the likelihood of acute MI. Lee et al. examined multiple chest pain characteristics to identify patients at low risk for acute MI. The combination of three variables – sharp or stabbing pain, no history of angina or acute MI, and pain that was pleuritic, positional, or reproducible – defined a very low-risk group [10]. Other studies have concluded that positional chest pain suggests a non-ACS etiology [11, 12]. Chest pain localized to a small area of the chest is often thought to suggest a musculoskeletal etiology. In one study, however, 27 of 403 patients (7%) with acute MI localized their pain to an area as small as a coin [13].

Chest wall tenderness, or reproducible chest pain, is a clinical feature that may persuade the EP to make a diagnosis of musculoskeletal pain. On examining the patient, the EP should be careful in determining if the pain induced by chest palpation is the same pain as the presenting pain. If there is no defined injury or event that could have led to a soft tissue injury, the EP should be reluctant to render a diagnosis of musculoskeletal pain.

> KEY FACT | 7% of patients with acute MI or unstable angina had their pain partially or fully reproduced on chest wall palpation.

Several studies have shown that chest wall tenderness can be misleading. In two separate studies, as many as 15% of patients diagnosed with acute MI had some degree of chest wall tenderness on examination [4, 14]. In another study, 17/247 (7%) of patients with acute MI or unstable angina had their pain partially or fully reproduced on chest wall palpation [10]. More recently, Disla et al. noted that 6% of patients with chest wall tenderness on their initial examination were ultimately diagnosed with acute MI [15].

Several other studies have demonstrated that chest wall tenderness "suggests" a non-ACS etiology of chest pain. In one prospective observational study, the presence of chest wall tenderness reduced the probability of acute MI (LR, 0.2; 95% CI, 0.1–1.0) [16]. Panju et al. and Chun and McGee concluded after separate meta-analyses that chest wall tenderness decreased the likelihood of acute MI (LR, 0.2–0.4; LR, 0.3 respectively) [17, 18]. However, considering the pre-test probability of acute MI noted in both meta-analyses (12.5–17.4%), the post-test probability of acute MI was still 4.3–6.3%.

Although certain chest pain characteristics decrease the likelihood of acute MI, none is powerful enough to support discharging at-risk patients without additional testing. In patients with chest pain, chest wall tenderness may suggest that acute MI is less likely but it does not effectively rule out the diagnosis. Given the potential implications of missing the diagnosis of acute MI, using chest wall tenderness as an independent rule out strategy is not recommended in patients at risk for ACS.

Pitfall | Assumption that acute MI cannot be diagnosed with a 12-lead ECG in the presence of pre-existing left bundle branch block or ventricular paced rhythm

The 12-lead ECG is an invaluable tool in the diagnosis of acute MI; in fact, it is the defining test of an ST-segment elevation MI (STEMI). There is a tendency to proffer diagnostic surrender when confronted with a patient presenting with signs and symptoms of ACS and an ECG that demonstrates either left bundle branch block (LBBB) or ventricular paced rhythm (VPR); the decision may be made to "wait for the cardiac enzymes" to establish a diagnosis. In fact, whereas these two electrocardiographic entities may confound or obscure the diagnosis of STEMI, there are published criteria that offer fairly specific (if not sensitive) evidence of STEMI in the face of LBBB and VPR.

LBBB
Delayed depolarization of ventricular myocardium in patients with LBBB results in the following characteristic findings:

1. QRS complex width > 0.12 s;
2. broad QS or rS pattern in the right precordial leads (leads V1, V2, and sometimes V3);

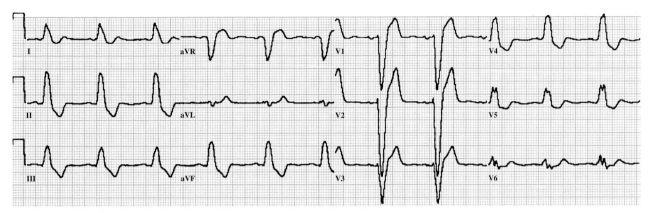

Figure 1.1 LBBB:
This tracing demonstrates an uncomplicated LBBB. Note the widened QRS complex (>0.12 s), the monophasic notched R-wave in the lateral leads (best seen in leads I and V5 here), and the absence of a Q-wave in lateral leads (I, aVL, V5, V6). There is discordance between the major vector of the QRS complex and the major vector of the ST-segment/T-wave complex that follows. Contrast these morphologies to those seen in Figure 1.2.

3. monophasic R-wave in the lateral leads (some, if not all, of leads I, aVL, V5, and V6); the absence of a q-wave in lateral leads.

Characteristically, in LBBB the affected leads also feature discordance of the ST-segment/T-wave complex: when the major QRS vector is directed downward (as in the right pre-cordial leads) the ST-segment will be elevated and the T-wave will be prominently positive. Similarly, if the major QRS vector is directed upward (as in the lateral leads), the ST-segment will be depressed and the T-wave will be inverted (see Figure 1.1). Loss of this characteristic pattern, often referred to as the "rule of appropriate discordance," is an electrocardiographic clue to acute MI in patients with LBBB.

> KEY FACT | ... STEMI can be diagnosed on an ECG with LBBB ... the ECG is more useful in ruling in the diagnosis than in excluding it.

Using the GUSTO-1 database, Sgarbossa and colleagues developed electrocardiographic criteria for STEMI in the face of pre-existing LBBB [19]. These criteria, listed in Table 1.2, can be committed to memory, but are perhaps better recalled after examining a tracing that demonstrates the criteria (see Figure 1.2) and comparing it to the appearance of LBBB without ischemia (see Figure 1.1). Meeting the threshold criterion score of ≥3 points (see Table 1.2) established the diagnosis of acute MI with 90% specificity. Others have reported problems with sensitivity and inter-rater reliability using the Sgarbossa criteria for acute MI in the presence of LBBB [20–22]. Smith and Whitwam argue that the sensitivity of the ECG for acute MI (as defined by CPK-MB elevation) *without* LBBB mirrors that of the ECG *with* LBBB – approximately 45% [23]. The important point to remember here is that the acute MI can be diagnosed on an ECG with LBBB, but that the ECG is more useful in ruling-in the diagnosis than in excluding it – just as

Table 1.2 Sgarbossa's criteria for STEMI in the presence of LBBB [19].

ST-segment elevation ≥1 mm concordant with QRS complex (score 5)
ST-segment depression ≥1 mm in leads V1, V2, or V3 (score 3)
ST-segment elevation ≥5 mm discordant to the QRS complex (score 2)

Score ≥3 means patient is likely experiencing a STEMI; score of <3 means ECG is indeterminate and more information is needed.

is the case in patients with symptoms of ACS and no LBBB (i.e., normal conduction) on their presenting ECG.

VPR

Returning to the GUSTO-1 database, Sgarbossa and colleagues generated electrocardiographic criteria for acute MI in the presence of a VPR [24]. Notably, these criteria were derived from an extremely small subject pool – 17 patients (as opposed to the 131 who had served a parallel role in the data set for LBBB and STEMI discussed above). The criteria that performed best were not surprisingly the same ones that were published for acute MI and LBBB [19]. However, the most useful criterion for acute MI in the presence of VPR was that which performed least well in the LBBB data set – STE ≥ 5 mm discordant to the QRS complex. Perhaps this is due to the fact that most ECGs with VPR feature very few principally positive QRS complexes; the vector generated by a ventricular pacing spike emanating from the right ventricular apex (where the pacing wire typically sits) results in predominantly negative QRS complexes in most if not all precordial leads and often in the inferior leads as well (see Figure 1.3). Thus, there is more "opportunity" to witness out-of-proportion discordant ST-segment elevation than there is to feature concordant ST-segment elevation or concordant ST-segment depression. However, both may be evident in acute MI in the presence of VPR (see Figure 1.4). And so, as with acute MI and LBBB, the ECG in the presence of VPR is more likely to rule in the diagnosis of acute MI than it is to rule it out.

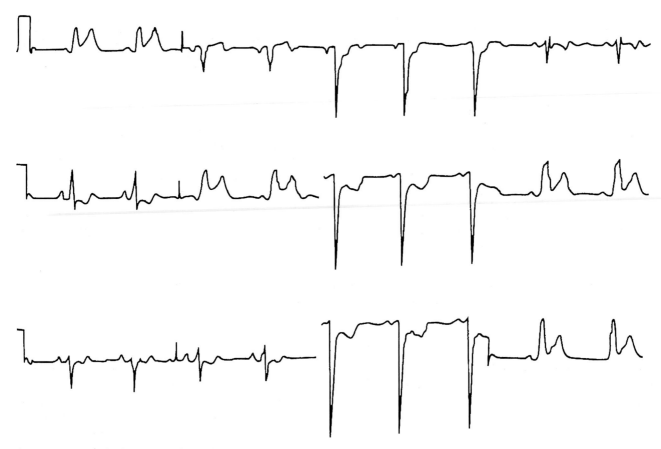

Figure 1.2 Acute MI in the presence of LBBB.

[Reproduced with permission from Elsevier; Brady WJ, Pollack ML. Acute myocardial infarction: confounding patterns. In: Chan TC, Brady WJ, Harrigan RA, et al. (eds). *ECG in Emergency Medicine and Acute Care*. Philadelphia: Elsevier Mosby, 2005, p. 183, Fig. 34-4.]. The ECG demonstrates concordant ST-segment elevation in leads I, aVL, V5, and V6 as well as concordant ST-segment depression in leads V1 to V3, violating the rule of appropriate discordance.

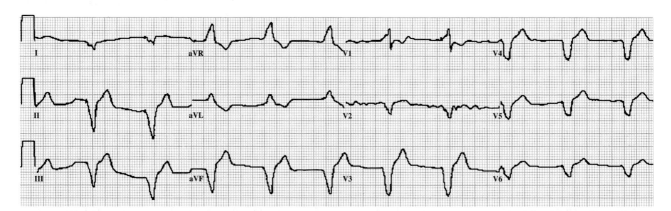

Figure 1.3 VPR:

This tracing shows a functioning ventricular pacemaker set at 60 bpm. Small-amplitude pacemaker spikes can be seen before the widened QRS complexes (these are best seen in leads II and V1 here). Note the predominance of negatively deflected QRS complexes – since 9 of 12 leads have negative QRS complexes, there is less opportunity for concordant ST-segment elevation – the criterion that functioned best in the study defining criteria for detection of acute MI with coexistent LBBB [19]. There is ample opportunity for the detection of discordant ST-segment elevation ⩾ 5 mm, however; this is the criterion that performed best in the study which defined criteria for detection of acute MI with coexistent VPR [24]. There is no evidence of acute MI on this tracing, however.

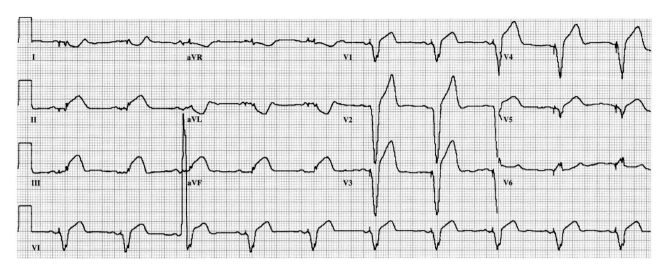

Figure 1.4 Acute MI in the presence of VPR.
[Reproduced with permission from Elsevier; Brady WJ, Pollack ML. Acute myocardial infarction: confounding patterns. In: Chan TC, Brady WJ, Harrigan RA, et al. (eds). *ECG in Emergency Medicine and Acute Care*. Philadelphia, Elsevier Mosby, 2005, p. 187, Fig. 34-10.]. The electrocardiogram demonstrates evidence of concordant ST-segment elevation in leads II, III, and aVF; and reciprocal ST-segment depression in leads I and aVL.

Pitfall | Use of a "GI cocktail" to distinguish between cardiac versus non-cardiac chest pain

Distinguishing gastroesophageal pain from ischemic chest pain can be difficult. Both may share similar characteristics such as dyspepsia and response to nitrates; however, one is an emergency and the other is not. A "GI cocktail" is sometimes used in the ED in an attempt to make this differentiation. Compositions vary, but a GI cocktail usually consists of a mixture of a liquid antacid, viscous lidocaine, and a liquid anticholinergic/barbiturate compound [25].

In one small study from the 1970s, Schwartz noted that the administration of a GI cocktail was highly reliable in differentiating ischemic chest pain from gastroesophageal pain. Sixty patients presenting with chest pain, epigastric pain, or both were treated with 20 ml of viscous lidocaine. None of the patients who obtained significant pain relief from the GI cocktail (37/60) were found to have myocardial ischemia. Among those who did not respond to the GI cocktail (23/60), myocardial ischemia or acute MI was diagnosed in more than half (13/23) [26].

More recently, Wrenn et al. performed a retrospective review of ED charts to determine the practice patterns regarding the administration of GI cocktails. During a 3-month period, 97 patients received a GI cocktail for various presenting complaints including abdominal pain (49), chest pain (40), and dyspnea (4). Over two-thirds of the patients (66/97) also received at least one other medication and the median time of administration of the other drug was 9 min before the GI cocktail. The most common medications given included opiates (56), nitroglycerin (22), and aspirin (10). Of the patients admitted for possible myocardial ischemia,

8/11 (73%) were noted to have some degree of relief after administration of a GI cocktail [27].

Beyond the research of Schwartz and Wrenn, the literature on the use of GI cocktails in the evaluation of chest pain is sparse. In one small case series, three patients diagnosed with acute MI had complete relief of their pain after administration of a GI cocktail [28]. One patient, however, did receive nitroglycerin in parallel with the GI cocktail. In another slightly larger case series, 7% of patients with ischemic chest pain got relief of their symptoms after receiving a GI cocktail [29].

Research on the use of the GI cocktail as a diagnostic test in the evaluation of chest pain is clearly limited. In addition, the interpretation of this test remains difficult because the GI cocktail is often administered soon before or after the administration of other potential pain relievers. One thing is clear: there is not enough evidence to suggest that the response of a patient with chest pain to a GI cocktail should in any way direct the disposition decision.

Pitfall | Assumption that a normal ECG rules out cardiac ischemia

When working through the differential diagnosis of chest pain, it is often said that the patient cannot be having an MI if ECG is normal. This is not true; in fact, no historical complaint, physical finding, or ECG pattern has a negative predictive value of 100% for MI. The patient may be less likely to be experiencing an MI if the ECG is normal, but more is needed than a normal ECG to discard the diagnosis. Furthermore, when considering the ECG and the literature behind this topic, a "normal" ECG must be strictly defined; that is, the negative predictive value of a normal ECG differs from that of an ECG with non-specific changes.

> KEY FACT | **6.4% of all patients with acute MI had a normal ECG.**

Data from the Acute Cardiac Ischemia-Time Insensitive Predictive Instrument (ACI-TIPI) trial highlights this issue. In that study, 889/10,689 patients were diagnosed with acute MI (by creatine kinase (CK)); 19 of those 889 were mistakenly discharged to home. Seventeen of those 19 (90%) had either a normal (2) or a non-ischemic (15) ECG. Four risks for inappropriate discharge were culled from that data; women <55 years old, non-white race, dyspnea as a chief complaint, and a normal ECG [30]. Combining data from two large studies totaling nearly 12,000 patients, of which nearly 2000 had an acute MI (again defined by CK criteria), Smith and colleagues [31] describe a concerning incidence of acute MI in patients with non-specific, and even normal, ECGs. Four hundred forty-two patients had a *non-specific* ECG yet had an acute MI – meaning 22.5% of all patients with acute MI had a non-specific ECG, and 8.6% of all patients with a non-specific ECG ended up having an acute MI. The normal ECG lessened the likelihood of acute MI, but the numbers here were still impressive: 125 patients had a *normal* ECG yet had an acute MI – translating to 6.4% of all patients with acute MI had a normal ECG, and 3.4% of all patients with a normal ECG had an acute MI. Smith et al. stress several important issues with these studies. They were performed in the pre-troponin era; it is unclear if only initial ECGs were included; and these studies did not differentiate ongoing chest pain from a history of recent chest pain [31].

Singer and associates showed that the negative predictive value of a "normal" ECG for acute MI does not improve as time passes from symptom onset – which seems counterintuitive. Analyzing data from 526 patients, 104 (20%) of whom had acute MI, they restricted their study to the initial ECG, yet did not report if the ischemic symptoms were ongoing. They found that the ECG maintained a 93% negative predictive value for acute MI at 0–12 h after the onset of symptoms [32]. Here, a "normal" ECG included those with non-specific ST-segment/T-wave changes as well as isolated fascicular blocks, illustrating again that this literature is at time confusing, in that the serum biomarker used to define MI varies, as does the definition of a "normal" ECG. What is clear is that the EP must not regard a non-specifically abnormal, or even a normal, ECG as proof-positive that a given patient is not presenting with symptoms of acute MI. Furthermore, a discussion of this issue is notably without reference to the predictive ability of the ECG in excluding unstable angina. The literature discussed above does not include this entity, and due to a lack of a clear gold standard definition of unstable angina, this remains a murky area of concern.

Pitfall | **Discharge of patients after a single set of negative cardiac enzymes**

In recent years, the role of cardiac markers in the diagnosis and treatment of patients with chest pain and suspected ACS has evolved considerably. A recent consensus guideline of the European Society of Cardiology (ESC) and the American College of Cardiology (ACC) redefined acute MI and highlighted the central importance of cardiac markers [33].

> KEY FACT | **[Cardiac enzymes] can only detect myocardial cell death but not ischemia.**

Cardiac markers provide a non-invasive means of determining whether myocardial damage has occurred. When ischemia gives way to infarction, the myocardial cell membrane is disrupted and various chemical markers are released into the systemic circulation. The timing of the rise of each cardiac marker is variable. Myoglobin is elevated within 2–4 h after acute MI and rapidly returns to baseline. CK-MB begin rising in the 3–6 h range and falls below the acute MI range at about 2 days. Troponin also begins rising at about 3–6 h post-infarction and gradually returns to baseline over approximately 1 week. In the past, elevation of the CK-MB fraction (CK-MB) was considered the gold standard in diagnosing acute MI. More recently, the cardiac troponins (I or T) have become the preferred cardiac markers for identifying myocardial damage. Regardless of which cardiac enzyme is used, however, it is important to remember that these tests can only detect myocardial cell death but not ischemia.

Cardiac troponins are highly sensitive for the detection of myocardial injury. A single troponin measurement at the time of presentation, however, appears to have limited utility in ruling out acute MI. The sensitivity of a single isolated troponin has been reported to be anywhere from 4% to 100% [34]. Variation in test sensitivity is explained by the timing of the troponin testing. Longer symptom duration yields higher sensitivity. Serial testing, especially when performed at least 6 h after symptom onset, markedly improves the sensitivity of troponins for acute MI. The evidence supporting the use of cardiac troponins in the diagnosis of non-MI ACS is limited. In up to 33% of patients diagnosed with classic unstable angina, cardiac troponins may be slightly elevated [35]. Current thought is now that these "enzyme leaks" are likely caused by micro-infarcts. In patients with ACS, increased troponin levels appear to be an indicator of increased risk for acute MI and death [36].

Once considered the gold standard, CK-MB is outperformed by cardiac troponins in terms of both sensitivity and specificity for acute MI. The sensitivity of a single CK-MB determination in diagnosing acute MI is also dependent on the elapsed time from symptom onset. The overall sensitivity of a single isolated CK-MB has been reported to be anywhere from 14% to 100% [34]. If testing occurs within 3 h of symptom onset, the sensitivity of CK-MB is only 25–50%. After 3 h, the sensitivity is increased, ranging from 40% to 100%. Because CK-MB rises relatively quickly, serial testing, even over a relatively short time period, has been shown to increase the sensitivity considerably. In one study, a change in a 2-h CK-MB level had a sensitivity of 93.2% for acute MI [37].

Myoglobin is found in both skeletal and cardiac muscle, thereby limiting its specificity. Because myoglobin is rapidly released after myocardial injury, it has been identified as a potential early indicator of acute MI. The sensitivity of a single myoglobin at the time of presentation, however, has been noted to be as low as 21% [34]. Serial testing significantly improves the diagnostic utility of myoglobin. In one study, doubling of the level 1–2 h after the initial measurement was nearly 100% sensitive for the diagnosis of acute MI [38].

More recent studies have looked into the use of serial measurements of multiple markers. McCord et al. noted that when myoglobin and troponin were drawn at presentation and at 90 min, the sensitivity for acute MI was 96.9% and the negative predictive value was 99.6% [39]. Ng et al. reported similar results utilizing a three-marker approach and a 90-min accelerated pathway, reporting nearly 100% sensitivity and 100% negative predicative value for acute MI [40]. It is critical to remember, however, that cardiac enzymes will not be reliably elevated in the setting of cardiac ischemia.

> KEY FACT | **Single determinations of cardiac markers at the time of presentation appear to be inadequate to exclude the diagnosis of acute MI and provide no information about the possibility of cardiac ischemia.**

Ultimately, determining the disposition of patients with suspected ACS requires the EP to gather and interpret many pieces of information. The combined data from the history, physical, ECG, and cardiac markers should guide the EP in managing a patient with chest pain or suspected ACS. Single determination of cardiac markers at the time of presentation appears to be inadequate to exclude the diagnosis of acute MI and provides no information about the possibility of cardiac ischemia.

Pitfall | **Over-reliance on a "classic" presentation for diagnosis of AD**

Acute dissection of the thoracic aorta is, unfortunately, both challenging to diagnose and potentially lethal if the diagnosis is missed. Furthermore, misattributing the chest pain of acute AD to ACS can lead to disastrous results as anticoagulant and fibrinolytic therapy are staples of the treatment of

the latter [41, 42]. Classically, the patient with AD has a history of hypertension and experiences the sudden onset of profound ripping or tearing chest pain that radiates to the back (interscapular region – perhaps migrating to the low back) [43]. It is important to note, however, that the absence of this history in no way excludes the diagnosis; symptoms may be atypical – or may even be absent. Indeed, one report [43] looking at pooled data from 16 studies, found a history of any pain to be only 90% sensitive for the diagnosis of acute AD (CI 85–94%) (see Table 1.3), with more precise and classic pain descriptions faring less well. Data reported from the International Registry of Acute Aortic Dissection (IRAD) [44] included 464 patients from 12 referral centers; some type of pain was reported in 94% of Type A dissections and 98% of Type B dissections; it was chest pain in 79% and 63%, respectively. The pain was abrupt in onset in roughly 85% of all dissections, and it was characterized as severe or the "worst ever" in 90% of both groups. Interestingly, it was classified as "sharp" (64%) more often than "ripping or tearing" (51%) [44]. Since the classic description has been well-documented to be less than universal, knowledge of atypical presentations of AD together with an awareness of risk factors enhances diagnostic capability.

Risk factors for AD [43].

- Hypertension
- Bicuspid aortic valve
- Previous cardiac surgery, particularly aortic valve replacement
- Coarctation of the aorta
- Marfan syndrome
- Ehlers–Danlos syndrome
- Turner syndrome
- Giant cell arteritis
- Third-trimester pregnancy
- Cocaine abuse
- Trauma

Table 1.3 Sensitivity of clinical history of pain in acute thoracic AD [43].

Pain Description	Sensitivity (%)	Confidence Intervals (%)
Any pain	90	85–94
Chest pain	67	56–77
Anterior chest pain	57	48–66
Posterior chest pain	32	24–40
Back pain	32	19–47
Abdominal pain	23	16–31
Sudden-onset pain	84	80–89
Severe pain	90	88–92
Ripping/tearing pain	39	14–69

So how do patients with acute AD present, if not with chest pain, or indeed any pain? *Syncope* was reported in 13% of Type A AD in IRAD; 2% of those patients did not have any pain or neurological findings (only 4% of Type B dissections presented with syncope) [44]. Others have reported syncope (at times painless) in acute AD as well [42, 45–47]. Another common diagnosis associated with acute AD is *acute stroke*, this being mediated by flap occlusion of a carotid artery in Type A dissection. IRAD data found 17/289 (6%) to present with acute stroke symptoms [44]; the more broadly defined finding of a new focal neurologic deficit was reported in 17% of pooled studies [43]. The neurologic deficit may be peripheral rather than central, due to the site of occlusion; motor and sensory findings in a lower extremity have been reported with acute AD in the absence of pain [48]. AD may also present as an acutely painful ischemic leg or as acute chest pain radiating to the back with simultaneous incontinence and bilateral lower extremity paralysis. Other atypical presentations of acute AD include abdominal or flank pain, hoarseness (recurrent laryngeal nerve compression), swelling and bruising of the neck, cough (mainstem bronchus compression), dysphagia (esophageal compression), Horner's syndrome (sympathetic chain compression), pulsatile sternoclavicular joint, superior vena cava syndrome, and testicular/groin pain [43–46, 49–51].

Pitfall | Use of the chest X-ray to exclude the diagnosis of AD

AD is the most common fatal condition involving the aorta [45]. Left untreated, about 75% of patients with AD involving the ascending aorta will die within 2 weeks. If diagnosed early and treated successfully, the 5-year survival rate approaches 75% [49]. Because early diagnosis is so important, the EP must maintain a high level of suspicion for AD. In the setting of chronic hypertension, AD should be considered in any patient with sudden and severe chest or back pain.

When AD is being considered, a chest X-ray should be obtained and examined for abnormalities of the aortic silhouette. This is best accomplished with a standing posteroanterior (PA) view. Portable anteroposterior (AP) views may falsely enlarge the cardiomediastinal silhouette and lateral chest X-rays rarely show evidence of AD [52]. Many radiographic findings have been noted in AD but unfortunately the majority of these findings are subjective and not well defined. Although the chest X-ray may suggest the diagnosis, it is rarely definitive.

Radiographic findings in AD may include widening of the mediastinum, abnormalities of the aortic knob and aortic contour, increased aortic diameter, left-sided pleural effusion, tracheal deviation, and esophageal deviation [49, 53]. The double density sign is observed when the false lumen is less radiopaque than the true lumen [49]. The calcium sign, consisting of the displacement of the aorta's intimal calcification

from the aortic knob by 1 cm or more, is highly suggestive of AD but is only present in a minority of cases [43, 49].

Widened mediastinum, defined as a measurement ≥ 8 cm at the level of the aortic knob, is considered by many to be the most sensitive radiographic finding. According to one study, widening of the mediastinum and widening of the aortic knob were the only two radiographic features of significance in predicting dissection [54]. A tortuous aorta, common in hypertensive patients, may widen the mediastinum and be hard to distinguish from AD. Other causes of mediastinal widening include adenopathy, lymphoma, and an enlarged thyroid.

> KEY FACT | **A widened mediastinum was noted in only 62% of all patients and an abnormal aortic contour was noted in only 50% of all patients.**

The IRAD, consisting of 12 international referral centers, published data on 464 patients diagnosed with AD. A widened mediastinum was noted in only 62% of all patients and an abnormal aortic contour was noted in only 50% of all patients (see Table 1.4). However, 21.3% of the patients were noted to have an absence of both a widened mediastinum and an abnormal aortic contour and 12.4% did not have any abnormalities noted on their chest X-rays [44].

In a meta-analysis of 13 studies, which included 1337 radiographs of patients diagnosed with AD, the sensitivity of plain chest X-rays was noted to be 90%. Absence of a widened mediastinum and abnormal aortic contour, in particular, decreased the probability of disease (negative LR, 0.3; 95% CI, 0.2–0.4). However, no specific radiographic abnormality was dependably present and therefore the absence of any one particular finding could not be used to rule out AD [43].

When asked to evaluate the presenting chest X-ray of patients with and without AD in a blinded manner, physicians from various specialties read 84% of the normal films as "not suspicious" for AD and only 73% of the AD films as "suspicious" for AD [55]. The most frequent finding identified on the AD chest X-rays was a widened mediastinum (38%). In another study, EP read 32% of AD chest X-rays as

Table 1.4 Chest X-ray findings in AD (Types A and B) [44].

Radiographic Finding	% Present
No abnormalities	12
Absence of widened mediastinum or abnormal aortic contour	21
Widened mediastinum	62
Abnormal aortic contour	50
Abnormal cardiac contour	26
Pleural effusion	19
Displacement/calcification of aorta	14

"normal" and noted a widened mediastinum only 10% of the time [45].

Although an apparently normal chest X-ray may decrease the likelihood of AD, it cannot be used exclusively to rule out the diagnosis of AD. If the clinical history and/or physical examination raise the suspicion for AD, further imaging should always be pursued.

Pitfall | Over-reliance on the presence of classic pleuritic chest pain and dyspnea in the evaluation of PE

PE remains a common cause of morbidity and mortality. Because so many cases of PE go undiagnosed, the actual incidence of PE remains unknown. Most cases of fatal PE are not actually diagnosed until autopsy. Despite advances in diagnostic methods and treatment over the last several decades, mortality rates have changed very little [56].

When promptly diagnosed and treated, PE rarely causes death. In fact, less than 10% of deaths caused by PE occur in those patients in which treatment is initiated. The majority of deaths (90%) occur in patients who are never treated because the diagnosis is never made [57].

The clinical presentation of PE is often subtle and many patients may actually be asymptomatic. The true rate of asymptomatic PE in the general population is unknown. In one study, of 387 patients diagnosed with PE, 34% of the patients were asymptomatic [56]. Atypical presentations may also occur. Patients may present with non-pleuritic chest pain, abdominal pain, back pain, fever, cough, wheezing, palpitations, and syncope [56, 58].

The classic triad of pleuritic chest pain, dyspnea, and hemoptysis is not only non-specific but it is also not sensitive. At most it is present 20% of the time [58]. The combination of chest pain, dyspnea, and tachypnea has been noted be as high as 97% sensitive for PE in various studies. However, the patients enrolled in these studies had symptoms suggestive of PE. Thus, patients with atypical features and asymptomatic patients were excluded [56].

> KEY FACT | **The presence of pleurisy is neither sensitive nor specific for PE. In one study … pleuritic chest pain occurred in only 44% of patients with PE versus 30% of patients without PE.**

Pleuritic chest pain has long been considered one of the classic symptoms of PE. However, its presence is neither sensitive nor specific for PE. In one study, for example, pleuritic chest pain occurred in only 44% of patients with PE versus 30% of patients without PE. In fact, the pain was described instead as substernal chest pressure, typical of cardiac ischemia, in 16% [59]. Chest pain is more common if pulmonary infarction has occurred because of pleural irritation.

Pulmonary infarction is more likely to occur in older patients with underlying cardiopulmonary disease [58]. In one study, nearly three quarters of patients with proven PE had pulmonary infarction [56].

Patients with PE are more likely to report dyspnea. In one study, sudden onset of dyspnea was by far the most frequent symptom in patients with PE, occurring in nearly 80% of the patients diagnosed with PE [59]. In another study, as many as 92% of patients diagnosed with PE reported dyspnea [60]. However, the severity of dyspnea is not always related to the degree of obstruction within the pulmonary vasculature. It has been suggested that many patients can be asymptomatic with as much as a 50% obstruction [61].

The signs and symptoms of PE are relatively non-specific and therefore the clinical recognition of PE is difficult. Although pleuritic chest pain and dyspnea make the diagnosis of PE more likely, the absence of these symptoms should not rule out the diagnosis.

Pitfall | The use of ECG findings to rule in or rule out PE

Patients with PE typically present with some combination of dyspnea, chest pain, tachypnea, and tachycardia – yet as with most illnesses, there is no combination of findings on the history and physical examination that either clinches or excludes the diagnosis. Thus, the EP looks to other easily obtainable tests (e.g., ECG, chest X-ray, D-dimer assay) when confronted with a patient with these signs and symptoms. The $S_1Q_3T_3$ pattern on ECG has long been linked with the diagnosis of PE, yet the literature suggests it is neither sensitive nor specific for PE.

Roughly 70 years ago, the $S_1Q_3T_3$ pattern was first reported in a series of seven patients with acute right heart strain secondary to PE, and was defined as such: an S-wave in lead I and a Q-wave in lead III with an amplitude of at least 0.15 mV (1.5 mm), and an associated inverted T-wave in lead III [62]. Others have avoided a strict criterion amplitude for these findings, or have used a variation of this finding, when looking at the ECG in PE [59, 63, 64]. Combining their data with those of three other studies, Ferrari and colleagues found the incidence of $S_1Q_3T_3$ to range from 12% to 50% in patients with *confirmed* PE [65]. Others stress the importance of looking at the incidence of a finding (such as $S_1Q_3T_3$) in patients with *suspected* PE (which generalizes more readily to our situation in the ED, where we are seeking a diagnosis) – where it has been found with equivalent frequency (approximately 12%) in patients with and without PE [66]. In either patient population, the $S_1Q_3T_3$ pattern is clearly not sensitive or specific for PE.

> KEY FACT | **Sinus tachycardia was found in only 8–69% of patients (with PE).**

Another ECG finding that is classically linked with PE – sinus tachycardia – should be recognized as less than universal; sinus tachycardia was found in only 8–69% of patients over six studies [67]. Other electrocardiographic findings occur at relatively low rates as well, including right atrial strain (2–31%) and right bundle branch block (6–67%) [67]. There are scattered reports of other entities, including atrial fibrillation and flutter, new changes in frontal plane QRS axis (especially rightward shift), clockwise shift in the precordial transition zone (i.e., toward the left precordial leads), low QRS voltage, ST-segment depression, and $S_1S_2S_3$ [63, 67, 68].

> KEY FACT | **Precordial T-wave inversion was the most common finding, occurring in 68% of patients with confirmed PE.**

So what ECG finding, if any, should be linked with PE? Ferrari [65] found precordial T-wave inversion was the most common finding in their series of 80 patients, occurring in 68% of patients with confirmed PE. The frequency of this finding exceeded those of sinus tachycardia (26%) and $S_1Q_3T_3$ (50%) in their series.

Two points should be emphasized with regard to this topic. First, the literature on the incidence of any ECG finding in PE comes principally from populations where the people are known to have the disease – thus they may have more obvious disease (i.e., large PEs) since they entered the subject pool when someone made the diagnosis. Second, ECG changes that resemble cardiac ischemia, especially T-wave inversions, can occur in patients with PE. Physicians should never rule in or rule out PE simply based on ECG finding.

Pitfall | **Failure to differentiate pericarditis from other chest syndromes**

On the surface, pericarditis seems as though it would be easy to recognize. Classically, pericarditis features the rather sudden onset of progressive, central, pleuritic chest pain that is worse with lying supine and improved with sitting up and leaning forward. On physical examination, a mono-, di-, or tri-phasic pericardial friction rub will be heard best when the patient is sitting up and leaning forward. The ECG shows diffuse ST-segment elevation, usually with PR-segment depression, while lead aVR (due to its opposite vector polarity) often demonstrates PR-segment elevation with ST-segment depression [69]. In actuality, however, acute pericarditis may be the great masquerader, in that historical features may vary, the elusive rub may be difficult to capture with the stethoscope, and the ECG bears some similarity to other syndromes, most notably ACS and benign early repolarization (BER).

Confusingly, pericarditis shares historical characteristics with other diseases such as pleurisy, PE, pneumothorax, pneumonia, acute MI, AD, and chest wall pain. All may feature pleuritic chest pain; the location of the pleural irritation may localize the pain away from the heart, moving other diagnoses up on the differential hierarchy. Proximal AD may be complicated by the development of a pericardial effusion, as might pericarditis – thus sudden onset of chest pain plus pericardial effusion on bedside ultrasound does not necessarily equal either disease. Like acute MI, the chest pain in pericarditis may radiate to the neck or shoulder area; however, radiation to the trapezius ridge(s) suggests pericarditis, because both phrenic nerves course through the anterior pericardium and innervate each trapezius ridge [69, 70]. Thus, the history is important but often insufficient in distinguishing the cause of the pain.

How often a pericardial rub is detectable in acute pericarditis is really not known; rubs are notoriously transient and unpredictable, although if present, they are virtually pathognomonic for pericarditis [69, 71, 72]. Rubs vary in description (e.g., rasping, creaking, scraping, grating, scratching, squeaking) and seem to overlie normal heart sounds. Typically best heard along the mid-to-lower left sternal border, rubs are best accentuated by positioning that brings the heart closer to the anterior chest wall – sitting up and leaning forward, or examination of the patient on all fours [70–72]. Experts differ on which phase of respiration optimizes auscultation of the rub – end-expiration [70, 72] or inspiration (if there is increased pericardial fluid) [71]. Pleural rubs are best distinguished from pericardial ones by location and phasic variation – the former varies with breathing, the latter with the heart cycle [70, 72]. If three phases occur with a pericardial rub, they are attributed to atrial systole, ventricular systole, and early diastolic filling [70, 71]. Signs of pericardial tamponade – hypotension, tachycardia, elevated jugular venous distension, muffled heart sounds, pulsus paradoxus – should be sought; however, these will be absent in pericarditis without sufficient effusion to cause or approach tamponade physiology. Tamponade may be expected in approximately 15% of cases of idiopathic origin, and as many as 60% of cases due to neoplastic, purulent, or tuberculous causes [70].

It is important to realize that laboratory diagnosis offers another juncture for confusion in this disease. Elevation of the peripheral leukocyte count, sedimentation rate, and C-reactive protein are neither sensitive nor specific. Disturbingly, serum troponin levels are elevated in 35–50% of patients – due to either epicardial inflammation or, more rarely, myocardial involvement in the form of myocarditis. Serum troponin elevation varies directly with the magnitude of ST-segment elevation on the ECG [70, 73]. Thus, three hallmarks of acute MI – chest pain radiating to the neck and shoulder, elevation of serum troponin, and ST-segment elevation on the ECG – may be seen with pericarditis. With that being said, the subtleties of the ST-segment elevation are usually helpful in distinguishing the two diseases.

ST-segment elevation, at times subtle and at times pronounced, can be seen in both acute MI and acute pericarditis.

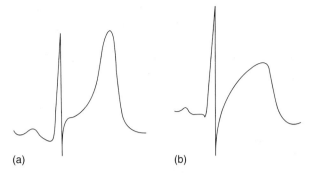

Figure 1.5 ST-segments in acute pericarditis and acute MI. [Reproduced with permission from Elsevier; Chan, TC. Myopericarditis. In: Chan TC, Brady WJ, Harrigan RA, et al. (eds). *ECG in Emergency Medicine and Acute Care*. Philadelphia: Elsevier Mosby, 2005, p. 203, Fig. 37-7.]. (a) demonstrates concave ST-segment elevation typical of acute pericarditis. Acute MI may also demonstrate this same type of ST-segment morphology. However, the presence of concurrent PR-segment depression confirms the diagnosis of acute pericarditis; (b) demonstrates convex ST-segment elevation highly specific for acute MI.

Morphologically, the ST-segments of acute pericarditis are classically concave upward, whereas the ST-segments in acute MI can be concave upward, straight, or convex upward (see Figure 1.5) [74]. One morphologic feature of the ST-segment that distinguishes acute MI from pericarditis is reciprocal ST-segment depression; with the former, this dramatically increases the specificity of the ECG. Reciprocal ST-segment depression may logically appear on the ECG in the area representing the opposing electrical view from that of the infarcted territory; for example, in inferior (leads II, III, and aVF) STEMI, lead aVL (which is directed 150° opposite to lead III in the frontal plane) may demonstrate ST-segment depression (which also may be seen, to a lesser extent, in lead I) [75]. Save for lead aVR and at times lead V1, the presence of ST-segment depression on the ECG in acute pericarditis is extremely rare [71, 75, 76]. This emphasizes another key distinction on the ECG between acute MI and pericarditis – the former features regional abnormalities that reflect infarct territory of the affected coronary artery, whereas most cases of acute pericarditis demonstrate diffuse ST-segment elevation. Similarly, regional development of Q-waves in the company of ST-segment elevation favors acute MI [72, 75].

PR-segment depression is another distinguishing feature of the ECG in acute pericarditis. As with ST-segment changes, diffuse changes suggest pericarditis; focal, regional changes do not. PR-segment depression is itself of undetermined specificity, and can be seen in atrial infarction. Leads II, V5, and V6 often feature the most obvious PR-segment depression; lead aVR may again behave oppositely, revealing PR-segment elevation in acute pericarditis. PR-segment depression may coincide with or even precede ST-segment elevation in pericarditis [69, 71, 72, 76]. PR-segment depression is most specific for acute pericarditis when it occurs in multiple leads; however, the finding is transient and is therefore not universally present in all patients with pericarditis.

> KEY FACT | **T-waves do not invert in pericarditis until the resolution of the ST-segment elevation phase, whereas in acute MI, they may invert while the ST-segments remain elevated.**

Like the PR- and ST-segments, the T-wave behaves differently in acute MI and pericarditis. While both diseases can feature T-wave inversions following ST-segment elevation, there is an important distinction: T-waves do not invert in pericarditis until the resolution of ST-segment elevation phase, whereas in acute MI, they many invert while the ST-segments remain elevated [70, 77]. This characteristic serves to emphasize the value of serial ECG sampling; regional ST-segment evolution, and the timing of dynamic T-wave changes will aid in securing a diagnosis.

Stepping away from the electrocardiographic similarities and differences of acute MI and pericarditis, some attention must be given to differentiating acute pericarditis from BER on the ECG – should a patient with baseline BER on the ECG present with chest pain consistent with pericarditis. Both pericarditis and BER feature diffuse ST-segment elevation with concave upward morphology. Marked PR depression may occur in pericarditis, whereas mild PR depression, as a function of the natural process of atrial depolarization [75], may be seen on any ECG, including those with BER. One useful distinguishing factor is that the ST-segment elevation of BER is stable over time (i.e., should be present on old tracings), whereas the ST-segment elevation of acute pericarditis, though not given to minute-to-minute change (unlike ACS), should be absent on old ECGs, should they be available for comparison [78]. Another useful distinguishing characteristic focuses on the relative amplitudes of the J point and the T-wave. If the height of the J point in lead V6 measures more than 25% of the amplitude of the corresponding T-wave peak, the ECG diagnosis is likely pericarditis, rather than BER. The end of the PR-segment should be used as a baseline when making this comparison [79, 80]. Restated, pericarditis yields more ST-segment elevation per T-wave amplitude (in lead V6) than does BER (see Figure 1.6).

Pericarditis can be difficult to diagnose – with similarities to other diseases in history, laboratory test results, and electrocardiographic appearance. The evidence must be weighed in total in difficult cases. Furthermore, a case can be made for urgent echocardiography as a diagnostic adjunct. Since any form of pericardial inflammation can lead to pericardial effusion, echocardiography is recommended when making the diagnosis of pericarditis [69]. Thus, the degree of effusion can be assessed, which has important implications for treatment and disposition. Moreover, regional wall motion abnormalities may be seen in acute MI, whereas they would not be expected (unless pre-existing) in pericarditis or BER. Echocardiography is also the best test to detect ventricular aneurysm, which also may cause ST-segment elevation on the ECG [81].

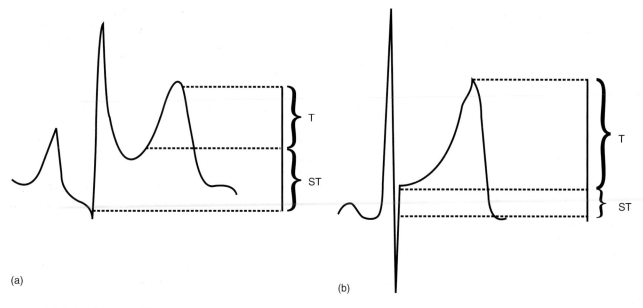

(a)

(b)

Figure 1.6 Pericarditis versus BER.

Acute pericarditis and BER can be differentiated on the ECG by determining the ratio of the ST segment and T wave amplitudes. The terminal portion of the PR segment should be used as the baseline for the purpose of performing this calculation. Typically lead V6 is evaluated. A ratio (ST segment/T wave) of ⩾0.25 favors a diagnosis of pericarditis (a), whereas BER (b) is more likely if the ratio is <0.25. [79]

Pitfall | Assumption that the standard chest X-ray completely rules out pneumothorax

Pneumothorax is a common condition affecting all age groups. It may occur spontaneously or as the result of trauma. Primary spontaneous pneumothoraces most often occur in tall, young males without any underlying parenchymal lung disease. A history of smoking is very common (90%). Secondary spontaneous pneumothoraces occur in older patients with known lung disease, primarily chronic obstructive pulmonary disease (COPD). Depending on the severity of the underlying disease and the size of the pneumothorax, secondary spontaneous pneumothoraces can be life threatening. In fact, COPD patients have a 3.5 fold increase in mortality when spontaneous pneumothoraces occur. Tension pneumothorax in the absence of trauma is relatively rare, and is associated with spontaneous pneumothorax in only 1–3% of cases [82]. Traumatic pneumothoraces occur as the result of blunt or penetrating trauma or as complication of a medical procedure. Tension pneumothoraces are much more likely to develop in the setting of trauma.

The classic symptoms of pneumothorax include pleuritic chest pain and shortness of breath. However, nearly one-third of patients (30%) may be asymptomatic or present only with minor complaints [82]. On physical examination, there may be decreased chest wall movement, hyperresonance to percussion, and decreased or absent breath sounds on the affected side.

The chest X-ray is the primary diagnostic modality used to screen for pneumothorax. The overall sensitivity of chest X-rays in detecting pneumothorax has been reported to be as high as 80%. Diagnosis is typically made by identifying a visceral pleural line on an upright, inspiratory chest X-ray. This line is seen initially at the apex of the lung and along the lateral pleural margin. The absence of lung markings peripheral to the pleural line may also be noted. With small pneumothoraces, an overlying rib may obscure the pleural line. Skin folds, the inner borders of the scapula, large bullae, and indwelling lines may all be mistaken for a pneumothorax. In most cases, an upright, inspiratory chest X-ray is the only study required to make the diagnosis.

If pneumothorax is strongly suspected and a pleural line is not visualized, an expiratory chest X-ray can be obtained. In full expiration the lung density is increased while the volume of air in the pleural space remains constant, in theory making it easier to detect a pneumothorax. A recent randomized controlled trial, however, revealed no difference in the ability of radiologists to detect pneumothoraces on inspiratory and expiratory films [83]. A lateral decubitus film can also be obtained. Although a lateral decubitus chest X-ray may be diagnostic, when clinically feasible, an upright chest X-ray is the procedure of choice for suspected pneumothoraces [84, 85].

Although the standard chest X-ray is usually sufficient to diagnose a pneumothorax, the literature demonstrates that missed pneumothoraces are still relatively common [85]. In 200 intensive care unit patients, 47 patients (23.5%) had missed pneumothoraces on routine chest X-rays [86]. In one study of 90 trauma patients, the initial supine chest X-ray failed to detect pneumothorax in 35 patients (39%) [87]. In another study of 103 severely injured patients with blunt trauma, 27 (26%) had pneumothoraces missed on their initial chest X-ray only to be picked up on thoracic CT [88]. In yet another study, one-third of all traumatic pneumothoraces were missed on the initial chest X-ray and diagnosed on abdominal CT [89]. If the initial chest X-ray is inconclusive and there is a significant suspicion of pneumothorax, CT imaging should be pursued in any high-risk patient group (COPD, trauma, mechanically ventilated). As the diagnostic sensitivity of a test (chest CT) increases, the issue of clinical relevance emerges. Clearly some trivial pneumothoraces found only on chest CT need no treatment.

Pitfall | Excluding the diagnosis of Boerhaave's syndrome due to an absence of antecedent retching or vomiting

First described by the Dutch physician Herman Boerhaave in 1724, Boerhaave's syndrome refers to rupture of the esophagus – and is associated with high morbidity and mortality. At times referred to as spontaneous rupture of the esophagus, Boerhaave's syndrome is probably best thought of as rupture due to the development of a tear after a rise in the intraluminal pressure of this structure. The classic triad for this syndrome includes forceful emesis, chest pain, and subcutaneous emphysema. Patients usually appear very ill, prefer to sit up and lean forward, and may have lateralizing pulmonary findings on examination (rales, wheezing, decreased breath sounds) in addition to the subcutaneous emphysema, if it is present. Chest X-ray abnormalities include atelectasis, infiltrates, and pleural effusion, usually on the left because 90% of cases are due to a tear in the left posterolateral wall of the lower third of the esophagus, which communicates with the left pleural cavity in 80% of cases. Pneumomediastinum and hydropneumothorax may be apparent on the chest X-ray as well. Definitive diagnosis is usually made by computed tomographic scan of the thorax or by esophagram, although false negative studies may occur with either [90–93].

> KEY FACT | **Antecedent retching or vomiting was absent in 21% of cases of Boerhaave's syndrome … the diagnosis should not be excluded in the absence of this historical feature.**

In one literature review [90] antecedent retching or vomiting was absent in 21% of cases of Boerhaave's syndrome. Thus, it should be emphasized that the diagnosis should not be excluded in the absence of this historical feature. Indeed, Boerhaave's syndrome has been reported after a variety of events, some less dramatic than others. Belching [94], simply swallowing a sandwich [95], violent cough [96], defecation, childbirth, weight lifting, asthma attacks, seizures,

and blunt abdominal trauma [97, 98] have all been reported as precipitant events for Boerhaave's syndrome. It has been reported to complicate the vomiting associated with acute MI [99]. It should especially be considered in patients with chest pain after a recent esophageal endoscopic procedure. Notably, it is also seen in children [97, 98], and may present with a right-sided esophageal tear – leading to findings on physical examination and chest X-ray on the right side rather than the classic occurrence on the left [91, 98]. Thus, as with most diseases, atypical isolated features of the history and physical examination, and even negative initial diagnostic tests, should not dissuade the EP from pursuing the diagnosis of Boerhaave's syndrome if the patient appears ill and the diagnosis remains possible yet illusive.

Pitfall | Failure to evaluate a patient with chest tenderness for herpes zoster

We have all seen patients in a less-than optimal setting (e.g., in a chair; multiple layers of clothes on; no curtain for privacy) where we take the chest pain history and find that the pain is reproducible with palpation on physical examination. When entertaining the diagnosis of chest wall pain or costochondritis, consider herpes zoster (shingles) as well.

Herpes zoster is generally a clinical diagnosis. It occurs in patients due to reactivation of latent varicella zoster virus, dormant in the dorsal root ganglia. It is seen in both children and adults, although incidence varies directly with age [100, 101]. Annualized incidence is 1.5–3.0 case per 1000 persons; in patients >75 years of age, this rate increases to 10 cases per 1000 persons [100]. The increased incidence with age, as well as an association with states of impaired cell-mediated immunity (e.g., immunosuppressive therapy, cancer, human immunodeficiency virus) is evident, but an outbreak of herpes zoster is not specific for a state of impaired immunity [100, 102]. Indeed, herpes zoster develops in approximately 20,000 apparently healthy children each year in the USA; chicken pox at an age of less than 1 year is a risk factor [102].

Herpes zoster typically presents with abnormal skin sensations (itching, tingling, and/or pain – which may be severe) in a dermatomal distribution that precede the appearance of skin lesions – typically by 1–5 days [100], although visible lesions may not develop for a week to 10 days [103, 104]. *Zoster sine herpete* is an uncommon variant in which the lesions never appear [104]. The history together with visible evidence of the lesions (classically an erythematous maculopapular rash which progresses to the vesicular stage, followed by pustulation, ulceration, and finally crusting before disappearance) in a dermatomal distribution is key to the diagnosis [100]. Pain on light touch (allodynia) or overly sensitive skin (hyperesthesia) in a dermatomal distribution is also consistent with the diagnosis; these findings may precede the outbreak of the skin lesions [104]. Generally speaking, the rash is unilateral, does not cross the midline, and is confined to one dermatome in immunocompetent persons. Overlap with adjacent dermatomes is relatively common (20%), and the appearance of a few lesions outside the affected dermatome is also not unusual [100]. Resolution occurs over 2–4 weeks, although it may be followed by the persistence of pain – so-called post-herpetic neuralgia.

Thus, in patients with a presumptive diagnosis of chest wall pain, carefully inspect the skin for signs of herpes zoster. Furthermore, if no lesions are visible, but the history (pain, oftentimes severe, in a band-like, dermatomal distribution, and perhaps accompanied by itching or paresthesias) and physical examination (hyperesthesia or allodynia in the same dermatomal distribution) are consistent with the prodromal stage of herpes zoster, instruct the patient to watch carefully for the appearance of any lesions. Prompt treatment (generally within 3 days of appearance of the rash) with antiviral therapy is indicated [100].

Pearls for Improving Patient Outcomes

- Do not exclude the diagnosis of acute cardiac ischemia or MI based on the absence of pain, especially when evaluating diabetic patients, the elderly, and women.
- Never use reproducible chest wall tenderness to exclude the diagnosis of acute MI.
- When the ECG shows LBBB or VPR, examine it closely for signs of inappropriately large, discordant ST-segment elevation; concordant ST-segment elevation; or concordant ST-segment depression (in the right precordial leads) – these may indicate an acute MI.
- Never use the response to antacids as a diagnostic test for distinguishing cardiac versus gastric pain.
- Neither a single normal ECG nor a single negative set of cardiac enzymes should be used to rule out acute cardiac ischemia.
- The chest X-ray can be used to suggest the diagnosis of AD, but it cannot definitively exclude the diagnosis.
- Consider AD and PE in the differential diagnosis of patients presenting with syncope.
- Pleuritic chest pain should prompt diagnostic consideration of PE as well as acute pericarditis.
- Precordial T-wave inversions in patients with chest pain should prompt consideration of not only acute cardiac ischemia but also of acute PE.
- Boerhaave's syndrome should be considered in the differential diagnosis for all patients with chest pain, even in the absence of a history of retching or vomiting.
- Always visualize the skin whenever a patient has reproducible chest well tenderness, and look for evidence of herpes zoster.

References

1. Canto JG, Shlipak MG, Rogers WJ, et al. Prevalence, clinical characteristics, and mortality among patients with myocardial infarction presenting without chest pain. *J Am Med Assoc* 2000; 283:3223–9.
2. Dorsch MF, Lawrence RA, Sapsford RJ, et al. Poor prognosis of patients presenting with symptomatic myocardial infarction but without chest pain. *Heart* 2001; 86:494–8.
3. Gupta M, Tabas JA, Kohn MA. Presenting complaint among patients with myocardial infarction who present to an urban, public hospital emergency department. *Ann Emerg Med* 2002; 40:180–6.
4. Uretsky BF, Farquahr DS, Berezin AF, et al. Symptomatic myocardial infarction without chest pain: prevalence and clinical course. *Am J Cardiol* 1977; 40:498–503.
5. Bayer AJ, Chadha JS, Farag RR, et al. Changing presentation of myocardial infarction with increasing old age. *J Am Geriatr Soc* 1986; 34:263–6.
6. Lusiani L, Perrone A, Pesavento R, et al. Prevalence, clinical features, and acute course of atypical myocardial infarction. *Angiology* 1994; 45:49–55.
7. McSweeney JC, Cody M, O'Sullivan P, et al. Women's early warning symptoms of acute myocardial infarction. *Circulation* 2003; 108:2619–23.
8. Jacoby RM, Nesto RW. Acute myocardial infarction in the diabetic patient: pathophysiology, clinical course, and prognosis. *J Am Coll Cardiol* 1992; 20:736–44.
9. Boie ET. Initial evaluation of chest pain. *Emerg Med Clin N Am* 2005; 23:937–57.
10. Lee TH, Cook EF, Weisberg MC, et al. Acute chest pain in the emergency room. Identification and examination of low risk patients. *Arch Intern Med* 1985; 145:85–9.
11. Lee TH, Rouan GW, Weisberg MC, et al. Clinical characteristics and natural history of patients with acute myocardial infarction sent home from the emergency room. *Am J Cardiol* 1987; 60:219–24.
12. Solomon CG, Lee TH, Cook EF, et al. Comparison of clinical presentation of acute myocardial infarction in patients older than 65 years of age to younger patients: the Multicenter Chest Pain Study experience. *Am J Cardiol* 1989; 63:772–6.
13. Swap CJ, Nagurney JT. Value and limitations of chest pain history in the evaluation of patients with suspected acute coronary syndromes. *J Am Med Assoc* 2005; 294:2623–9.
14. Tierney WM, Roth BJ, Psaty B, et al. Predictors of myocardial infarction in emergency room patients. *Crit Care Med* 1985; 13:526–31.
15. Disla E, Rhim HR, Reddy A, et al. Costochondritis: a prospective analysis in an emergency department setting. *Arch Intern Med* 1994; 154:2466–9.
16. Goodacre S, Locker T, Morris F, et al. How useful are the clinical features in the diagnosis of acute, undifferentiated chest pain? *Acad Emerg Med* 2002; 9:203–8.
17. Panju AA, Hemmelgarn BR, Gordon G, et al. Is this patient having a myocardial infarction? *J Am Med Assoc* 1998; 280:1256–63.
18. Chun AA, McGee SR. Bedside diagnosis of coronary artery disease: a systematic review. *Am J Med* 2004; 117:334–43.
19. Sgarbossa EB, Pinski SL, Barbagelata A, et al. Electrocardiographic diagnosis of acute myocardial infarction in the presence of left bundle branch block. *New Engl J Med* 1996; 334:481–7.
20. Shapiro NI, Fisher J, Zimmer GD, et al. Validation of electrocardiographic criteria for diagnosing acute myocardial infarction in the presence of left bundle branch block [Abstract]. *Acad Emerg Med* 1998; 5:508.

21. Shlipak MG, Lyons WL, Go AS, et al. Should the electrocardiogram be used to guide therapy for patients with left bundle branch block and suspected acute myocardial infarction? *J Am Med Assoc* 1999; 281:714–9.

22. Kontos MC, McQueen RH, Jesse RL, et al. Can MI be rapidly identified in emergency department patients who have left bundle branch block? *Ann Emerg Med* 2001; 37:431–8.

23. Smith SW, Whitwam W. Acute coronary syndromes. *Emerg Med Clin N Am* 2006; 53–89.

24. Sgarbossa EB, Pinski SL, Gates KB, et al. Early electrocardiographic diagnosis of acute myocardial infarction in the presence of ventricular paced rhythm. *Am J Cardiol* 1996; 77:423–4.

25. Welling LR, Waston WA. The emergency department treatment of dyspepsia with antacids and oral lidocaine. *Ann Emerg Med* 1990; 19:785–8.

26. Schwartz GR. Xylocaine viscous as aid in the differential diagnosis of chest pain. *JACEP* 1976; 5:981–3.

27. Wrenn K, Slovis CM, Gongaware J. Using the "GI cocktail": a descriptive study. *Ann Emerg Med* 1995; 26:687–90.

28. Servi RJ. Relief of myocardial ischemia pain with a gastrointestinal cocktail. *Am J Emerg Med* 1985; 3:208–9.

29. Bennett JR, Atkinson M. The differentiation between oesophageal and cardiac pain. *Lancet* 1966; 2:1123–7.

30. Pope JH, Aufderheide TP, Ruthazer R, et al. Missed diagnosis of acute cardiac ischemia in the emergency department. *New Engl J Med* 2000; 342:1163–70.

31. Smith SW, Zvosek DL, Sharkey SW, Henry TD (eds). *The ECG in Acute MI: An Evidence-based Manual of Reperfusion Therapy.* Philadelphia: Lippincott Williams & Wilkins, 2002, pp. 19–27.

32. Singer AJ, Brogan GX, Valentine SM, et al. Effect of duration from symptom onset on the negative predictive value of a normal ECG for exclusion of acute myocardial infarction. *Ann Emerg Med* 1997; 29:575–9.

33. The Joint European Society of Cardiology/American College of Cardiology Committee. Myocardial infarction redefined – a consensus document of the Joint European Society of Cardiology/American College of Cardiology Committee for the Redefinition of Myocardial Infarction. *J Am Coll Cardiol* 2000; 36:959–69.

34. Balk EM, Iaonnidis JP, Salem D, et al. Accuracy of biomarkers to diagnose acute cardiac ischemia in the emergency department: a meta-analysis. *Ann Emerg Med* 2001; 37:478–94.

35. Malasky BR, Alpert JS. Diagnosis of myocardial injury by biochemical markers: problems and promises. *Cardiol Rev* 2002; 10:307.

36. Antman EM, Tanasijevic MJ, Thompson B, et al. Cardiac specific troponin I levels to predict the risk of mortality in patients with acute coronary syndromes. *New Engl J Med* 1996; 335:1342–9.

37. Fesmire FM, Percy RF, Bardoner JB, et al. Serial creatine kinase (CK) MB testing during the emergency department evaluation of chest pain: utility of a 2-hour delta CK-MB of +1.6 ng/ml. *Am Heart J* 1998; 136:237–44.

38. Pope JH, Selker HP. Diagnosis of acute cardiac ischemia. *Emerg Med Clinic N Am* 2003; 21:27–59.

39. McCord J, Nowak RM, McCullough PA, et al. Ninety-minute exclusion of acute myocardial infarction by use of quantitative point-of-care testing of myoglobin and troponin I. *Circulation* 2001; 104:1483–7.

40. Ng SM, Krishnaswamy P, Morrisey R, et al. Ninety-minute accelerated critical pathway for chest pain evaluation. *Am J Cardiol* 2001; 88:611–7.

41. Marian AJ, Harris SL, Pickett JD, et al. Inadvertent administration of rtPA to a patient with type 1 aortic dissection and subsequent cardiac tamponade. *Am J Emerg Med* 1993; 11:613–5.

42. Davis DP, Grossman MD, Kiggins DC, et al. The inadvertent administration of anticoagulants to ED patients ultimately diagnosed with thoracic aortic dissection. *Am J Emerg Med* 2005; 23:439–42.

43. Klompas M. Does this patient have an acute thoracic aortic dissection? *J Am Med Assoc* 2002; 287:2262–72.

44. Hagan P, Nienaber CA, Isselbacher EM, et al. The International Registry of Acute Aortic Dissection (IRAD): new insights into an old disease. *J Am Med Assoc* 2000; 283:897–903.

45. Sullivan, PR, Wolfson AB, Leckey RD, Burke JL. Diagnosis of acute thoracic dissection in the emergency department. *Am J Emerg Med* 2000; 18:46–50.

46. Al-Hity W, Playforth MJ. Collapse, hoarseness of the voice and swelling and bruising of the neck: an unusual presentation of thoracic aortic dissection. *Emerg Med J* 2001; 508–9.

47. Young J, Herd AM. Painless acute aortic dissection and rupture presenting as syncope. *J Emerg Med* 2002; 22:171–4.

48. Beach C, Manthey D. Painless acute aortic dissection presenting as left lower extremity numbness. *Am J Emerg Med* 1998; 16:49–51.

49. Chen K, Varon J, Wenker OC, et al. Acute thoracic aortic dissection: the basics. *J Emerg Med* 1997; 15:859–67.

50. Chan-Tack KM. Aortic dissection presenting as bilateral testicular pain. *New Engl J Med* 2000; 343:1199.

51. Ashe A, Counselman FL. Acute thoracic aortic dissection [Letter]. *J Emerg Med* 2002; 23:301–2.

52. Smith DC, Jan GC. Radiological diagnosis of aortic dissection. In: Doroghazi RM, Slater EE (eds), *Aortic Dissection*. New York: McGraw-Hill, 1983, pp. 71–132.

53. Wheat MW. Pathogenesis of aortic dissection. In: Doroghazi RM, Slater EE (eds), *Aortic Dissection*. New York: McGraw-Hill, 1983, pp. 55–70.

54. Jagannath AS, Sos TA, Lockhart SH, et al. Aortic dissection: a statistical analysis of the usefulness of plain radiographic findings. *Am J Roentgenol* 1986; 147:1123–6.

55. Gregorio MC, Baumgartner FJ, Omari BO. The presenting chest roentgenogram in acute type A aortic dissection: a multidisciplinary study. *Am Surg* 2002; 68:6–10.

56. Ryu JH, Olson EJ, Pellikka PA. Clinical recognition of pulmonary embolism: problem of unrecognized and asymptomatic cases. *Mayo Clin Proc* 1998; 73:873–9.

57. Dalen JE. Pulmonary embolism: what have we learned since Virchow? Natural history, pathophysiology, and diagnosis. *Chest* 2002; 122:1440–56.

58. Laack TA, Goyal DG. Pulmonary embolism: an unsuspected killer. *Emerg Med Clin N Am* 2004; 22:961–83.

59. Miniati M, Prediletto R, Formichi B, et al. Accuracy of clinical assessment in the diagnosis of pulmonary embolism. *Am J Respir Crit Care Med* 1999; 159:864–71.

60. Susec O. The clinical features of acute pulmonary embolism in ambulatory patients. *Acad Emerg Med* 1997; 4:891–7.

61. Riedel M. Acute pulmonary embolism: 1. pathophysiology, clinical presentation, and diagnosis. *Heart* 2001; 85:229–40.

62. McGinn S, White PD. Acute cor pulmonale resulting from pulmonary embolism: its clinical recognition. *J Am Med Assoc* 1935; 104:1473–80.

63. Sreeram N, Cheriex EC, Smeets JLRM, et al. Value of the 12-lead electrocardiogram at hospital admission in the diagnosis of pulmonary embolism. *Am J Cardiol* 1994; 73:298–303.

64. Lualdi JC, Goldhaber SZ. Right ventricular dysfunction after acute pulmonary embolism: pathophysiological factors, detection, and therapeutic indications. *Am Heart J* 1995; 130:1276–81.

65. Ferrari E, Imbert A, Chevalier T, et al. The ECG in pulmonary embolism: predictive value of negative T waves in precordial leads – 80 case reports. *Chest* 1997; 111:537–43.

66. Rodger M, Makropoulos D, Turek M, et al. Diagnostic value of the electrocardiogram in suspected pulmonary embolism. *Am J Cardiol* 2000; 86:807–9.

67. Chan TC, Vilke GM, Pollack M, Brady WJ. Electrocardiographic manifestations: pulmonary embolism. *J Emerg Med* 2001; 21:263–70.

68. Manganelli D, Palla A, Donnamaria V, Giuntini C. Clinical features of pulmonary embolism: doubts and uncertainties. *Chest* 1995; 107:25S–32S.

69. Spodick, DH. Acute pericarditis. Current concepts and clinical practice. *J Am Med Assoc* 2003; 289:1150–3.

70. Lange R, Hillis LD. Acute pericarditis. *New Engl J Med* 2004; 351:2195–202.

71. Spodick DH. Pericardial diseases. In: Braunwald E, Zipes DP, Libby P (eds), *Heart Disease*, 6th ed. Philadelphia: W.B. Saunders, 2001, pp. 1823–71.

72. Troughton RW, Asher CR, Klein AL. Pericarditis. *Lancet* 2004; 363:717–27.

73. Bonnefoy E, Godon P, Kirkorian G, et al. Serum cardiac troponin I and ST-segment elevation in patients with acute pericarditis. *Eur Heart J* 2000; 21:832–6.

74. Smith SW. Upwardly concave ST segment morphology is common in acute left anterior descending coronary artery occlusion. *Acad Emerg Med* 2003; 10:516.

75. Smith SW, Whitwam W. Acute coronary syndromes: acute myocardial infarction and ischemia. In: Chan TC, Brady WJ, Harrigan RA, et al. (eds), *ECG in Emergency Medicine and Acute Care*. Philadelphia: Elsevier Mosby, 2005, pp. 151–72.

76. Chan TC. Myopericarditis. In: Chan TC, Brady WJ, Harrigan RA, et al. (eds), *ECG in Emergency Medicine and Acute Care*. Philadelphia: Elsevier Mosby, 2005, pp. 199–203.

77. Snider RL, Pai RK, Kusumoto FM. The importance of the evolution of the ST-T wave changes for differentiating acute pericarditis from myocardial ischemia. *Cardiology Rev* 2004; 12:138–40.

78. Brady WJ, Martin ML. Benign early repolarization. In: Chan TC, Brady WJ, Harrigan RA, et al. (eds), *ECG in Emergency Medicine and Acute Care*. Philadelphia: Elsevier Mosby, 2005, pp. 210–5.

79. Ginzton LE, Laks MM. The differential diagnosis of acute pericarditis from the normal variant: new electrocardiographic criteria. *Circulation* 1982; 65:1004–9.

80. Spodick DH. Electrocardiographic diagnosis of pericarditis [Reply]. *J Am Med Assoc* 2003; 289:2942–3.

81. Harper RJ. Ventricular aneurysm. In: Chan TC, Brady WJ, Harrigan RA, et al. (eds), *ECG in Emergency Medicine and Acute Care*. Philadelphia: Elsevier Mosby, 2005, pp. 213–5.

82. Weissberg D, Refaely Y. Pneumothorax: experience with 1199 patients. *Chest* 2000; 117:1279–85.

83. Seow A, Kazerooni EA, Pernicano PG, et al. Comparison of upright inspiratory and expiratory chest radiographs for detecting pneumothoraces. *Am J Roentgenol* 1997; 168:842–3.

84. Beres RA, Goodman LR. Pneumothorax: detection with upright versus decubitus radiography. *Radiology* 1993; 186:19–22.

85. Tocino IM, Miller MH, Fairfax WR. Distribution of pneumothorax in the supine and semirecumbent critically ill patient. *Am J Roentgenol* 1985; 144:901–5.

86. Lichtenstein DA, Meziere G, Lascols N, et al. Ultrasound diagnosis of occult pneumothorax. *Crit Care Med* 2005; 33:1231–8.

87. Bridges KG, Welch G, Silver M, et al. CT detection of occult pneumothorax in multiple trauma patients. *J Emerg Med* 1993; 11:179–86.

88. Trupka A, Waydhas C, Hallfeldt KJ, et al. Value of thoracic computed tomography in the first assessment of severely injured patients with blunt chest trauma: results of a prospective study. *J Trauma* 1997; 43:405–11.

89. Hill SL, Edmisten T, Holtzman G, et al. The occult pneumothorax: an increasing diagnostic entity in trauma. *Am Surg* 1999; 65:254–58.

90. Brauer RB, Libermann-Meffert D, Stein HJ, et al. Boerhaave's syndrome: analysis of the literature and report of 18 new cases. *Dis Esophagus* 1997; 10:64–8.

91. Rozycki GS. Image of the month (Esophageal perforation [Boerhaave's syndrome]) *Arch Surg* 2001; 136:355–6.

92. Bjerke HS. Boerhaave's syndrome and barogenic injuries of the esophagus. *Chest Surg Clin N Am* 1994; 4:819–25.

93. Atallah FN, Riu BM, Nguyen L, et al. Boerhaave's syndrome after postoperative vomiting. *Anesth Analg* 2004; 98:1164–6.

94. Sponk PE, Beishuizen A, van der Hoven B. Belching and the development of Boerhaave's syndrome. *Intens Care Med* 2001; 27:330.

95. Gopalan R, Cooke CG. Boerhaave's syndrome [Images in clinical medicine]. *New Engl J Med* 2000; 343:190.

96. Vyas H, Desai D, Abraham P, Joshi A. Heparin therapy for mistaken cardiac diagnosis in Boerhaave's syndrome. *Indian J Gastroenterol* 2004; 23:72–3.

97. Ramsook C. Boerhaave's syndrome: a pediatric case. *J Clin Gastroenterol* 2001; 33:77–8.

98. Kothari AA, Kothari KA. Atypical presentation of Boerhaave's syndrome. *Indian J Gastroenterol* 2004; 23:119.

99. Dominguez A, Garcia MJ, Rayo M, et al. Boerhaave's syndrome complicating acute myocardial infarction thrombolysis. *Intens Care Med* 2001; 27:1682.

100. Gnann JW, Whitley RJ. Herpes zoster. *New Engl J Med* 2002; 347:340–6.

101. Smith C, Glaser DA. Herpes zoster in childhood: case report and review of the literature. *Pediatr Dermatol* 1996; 13:226–9.

102. Feder HM. Herpes zoster [Letter]. *New Engl J Med* 2003; 348:2044–5.

103. Unger S, Lynfiedl Y, Alapati U. An atypical presentation of a common disease. *Arch Dermatol* 1998; 134:1279–84.

104. Montori VM, Rho J, Bauer BA. 37-year old man with back pain. *Mayo Clin Proc* 1999; 74:923–6.

Chapter 2 | Management of the Dyspneic Patient in the ED

Jairo I. Santanilla & Peter M. C. DeBlieux

Introduction

The American Thoracic Society consensus statement defines dyspnea as "a term used to characterize a subjective experience of breathing discomfort that consists of qualitatively distinct sensations that vary in intensity. The experience derives from interactions among multiple physiological, psychological, social, and environmental factors, and may induce secondary physiological and behavioral responses" [1]. This definition is broad and it shows the complex inter-relation of a patient's sensation, perception, and pathophysiology.

The mechanisms leading to dyspnea are not fully understood. They are multifactorial, complex, and involve many systems. The sensation of dyspnea is believed to originate in the insular cortex, a part of the limbic brain [2]. Chemoreceptors monitor the dynamic partial pressures of oxygen, carbon dioxide (CO_2), and pH. Mechanoreceptors in the airways, lung, and chest wall sense changes in pressure, flow, and volume in the pulmonary system. The respiratory complex, primary sensory cortex, primary motor cortex, chemoreceptors, mechanoreceptors, emotions, memories, and personality may directly and/or indirectly affect the insular cortex. The summation of this interplay is dyspnea.

Many patients will have several of the above mechanisms interacting when they complain of dyspnea. For example, patients in status asthmaticus have chemoreceptors stimulated by hypoxia and in later stages by hypercapnia. Mechanoreceptors will respond to decreased flow and hyperinflation. Both of these systems will stimulate the respiratory complex that will stimulate the lungs, chest wall, and insular cortex. The primary sensory cortex will sense the chest wall and lungs and activate the insular cortex. Finally, the sensation of dyspnea will be attenuated by the patient's level of fear, anxiety, and prior experiences.

Dyspnea has been shown to be an independent predictor of cardiovascular mortality [3]. In addition, patients suffering from dyspnea will use a multitude of descriptive terms; however, no single description can be used to exclude a disease process.

While the pathophysiology and differential diagnosis of dyspnea are quite intricate and daunting, we will attempt to provide some insight into several clinical scenarios that will lead to improved patient care. We will begin our discussion with pitfalls found in the physical examination and proceed through challenges with monitoring, imaging, laboratory tests, and treatment.

Pitfall | Relying on a normal physical examination to exclude disease

> KEY FACT | Positive physical examination findings should be used to modify the differential diagnosis. The absence of findings, however, should not be used to exclude disease as the sensitivity of examination findings for serious pathology is poor.

Traditionally, the importance of the history and physical examination is emphasized with great fervor to all medical students. Physical examination findings of a pneumothorax are taught as decreased breath sounds with hyper-resonance on percussion. Hirshberg et al. reported a case series of 51 patients with penetrating chest trauma with the conclusion that, "physical examination accurately predicted the need for tube thoracostomy with a sensitivity of 96% and a specificity of 93%" [4]. The detection of pneumothorax and hemopneumothorax on auscultation has been shown to have a positive predictive value of 97–98% [5, 6]. However, normal findings on the physical examination can miss significant pathology. More recent studies have shown that the sensitivity of auscultation ranges between 50% and 84% [5–7]. Factors such as pain, tenderness, or tachypnea are even less sensitive [7]. It is important to note that normal auscultory examinations have even been reported in cases of significant hemopneumothorax of up to 800 ml and 28% [6]. Relying solely on physical examination to exclude serious injury or illness is problematic. This has prompted many authors to recommend that all victims of penetrating trauma require chest radiographs because many will have hemopneumothorax in the absence of clinical findings [5, 7].

The accuracy and reliability of the physical examination is also called into question when considering the diagnosis of pneumonia and congestive heart failure (CHF). Wipf et al. describe physical examination to have a sensitivity of 47–69% and specificity of 58–75%, stating, "the traditional chest physical examination is not sufficiently accurate on its own to confirm or exclude the diagnosis of pneumonia" [8].

Other sources have also agreed that physical examination alone is insufficient to accurately diagnose pneumonia. There are no individual clinical findings, or combinations of findings, that have been found to accurately predict whether or not a patient has pneumonia [9]. Chakko et al. found that physical findings for patients with CHF (orthopnea, edema, rales, third heart sound, elevated jugular venous pressure) had poor predictive value for identifying patients with pulmonary capillary wedge pressure (PCWP) values greater than or equal to 30 mmHg [10].

Physical examination, particularly in the above examples, should be used to expand the differential diagnosis and should not be solely used to exclude disease in isolation. Instead, the physical examination should be used to broaden differential diagnoses when positive findings are present and should be used in conjunction with history and other clinical and radiographic studies.

Pitfall | Over-reliance on a normal pulse oximetry measurement

The use of pulse oximetry has become widespread over the past three decades. Most emergency physicians have quick and easy access to this "fifth" vital sign. Pulse oximetry has been used quite successfully to determine a patient's oxygenation status and it is very reliable in detecting hypoxia, especially in the arterial oxygen saturation range of 70–100%. However, over-reliance on normal pulse oximetry may lead to disastrous consequences in the critically ill, the chronically ill, or the over-sedated patient.

Pulse oximetry does not help determine the adequacy of a patient's ventilatory status. While pulse oximetry accurately detects hypoxia, it does not detect hypercapnia. Though some studies have suggested that it can screen for hypercarbia, these studies were in patients breathing room air, without supplemental oxygen. In addition, these same studies used a pulse oximetry of less than or equal to 96% as the cutoff [11, 12], limiting its utility in many patients presenting with dyspnea. Relying solely on pulse oximetry measures can become even more problematic when patients are receiving supplemental oxygen.

> KEY FACT | **While pulse oximetry is useful to identify patients with hypoxia, it does not identify patients with hypercarbia.**

There have been numerous reports of patients succumbing to hypercapnic respiratory failure while being maintained on supplemental oxygen and being monitored by continuous pulse oximetry. The danger of not detecting hypoventilation through pulse oximetry can be exemplified by the following cases: one inadvertently hypoventilated patient who was administered 100% oxygen during hip arthroplasty and monitored with pulse oximetry alone developed a $PaCO_2$ of 265 mmHg and an arterial pH of 6.65, despite maintenance of oxygen saturations of 94–96% [13]. Another patient, undergoing cosmetic facial surgery under general anesthesia, was ventilated by mask with an oxygen-enriched gas mixture for 4 to 6 h and monitored by pulse oximetry. Despite adequate arterial saturation ($SaO_2 > 90\%$) throughout the procedure, the patient remained in a deep coma after termination of anesthesia. Initial arterial blood gas analysis revealed a pH of 6.60 and a $PaCO_2$ of 375 mmHg [14]. These clinical examples are not far removed from procedural sedations that are routinely practiced in the emergency department (ED) for orthopedic and complex suturing procedures.

> KEY FACT | **The PaO_2 must decrease substantially before a change in the oxygen saturation will register via pulse oximetry.**

Another confounder on the impact of supplemental oxygen and pulse oximetry is that it requires a large drop in PaO_2 before the monitor detects a significant change. This confers a false sense of oxygenation reserve. For example, if a patient receives supplemental oxygen and the PaO_2 is 215 mmHg, the pulse oximeter will measure 100%. This reading will not change significantly until the PaO_2 drops to 65 mmHg before a decrease in oxygen saturation is detected [15].

Improper probe placement, ambient light, and sickle cell hemoglobin can all falsely elevate pulse oximetry readings, although this occurs rarely. Methemoglobinemia can provide either a falsely lower or elevated pulse oximetry measure depending on the percentage of methemoglobinemia. Carboxyhemoglobin, associated with CO poisoning, will produce a falsely elevated pulse oximetry reading that may mask potentially lethal desaturation [16]. Both toxidromes, when clinically significant, can present with shortness of breath and abnormal arterial blood gas, or carboxyhemoglobin results. Classically, venous blood samples in methemoglobinemia have a chocolate brown coloration and venous blood samples in carboxyhemoglobinemia offer a bright cherry red color.

The above noted inability of pulse oximetry to detect hypercapnia has lead to the development of other techniques of non-invasive monitoring. These devices fall under two categories; the first being end-tidal CO_2 detectors, and the second being combined pulse oximetry and CO_2 tension sensors. End-tidal CO_2 detectors have been shown to detect subclinical respiratory depression that was not detected by pulse oximetry alone [17]. In addition, combined sensors have been shown to correlate well with arterial measurements and have potential applications in the ICU, ED, sleep studies, and procedural sedation [18–20]. For procedural sedation emergency medicine physicians continue to use a multitude of anesthetic agents that suppress respiratory drives and have the potential to harm patients that possess limited cardiopulmonary reserve. To rely soley on pulse oximetry as a marker of respiratory effectiveness in this patient population is not prudent.

Pulse oximetry is a valuable tool in the evaluation of patients with dyspnea; however, it has limitations that should be kept in mind.

Pitfall | **Confusing dyspnea for anxiety**

While it is true that several psychiatric illnesses (most notably panic disorder) may have dyspnea as a feature, one must be careful not to take lightly the complaint of dyspnea in a psychiatric patient. Anxiety and depressive symptoms are common in elderly patients with chronic obstructive pulmonary disease (COPD). In addition the prevalence and severity of depressive symptoms may be greater in those who are most disabled [21]. There have been reports of a possible link between chronic dyspnea and suicide risk [22]. In addition, psychiatric disorders have been identified as risk factors for fatal or near-fatal asthma exacerbations [23]. Finally, in a Dutch study on the clinical presentation of acute myocardial infarct in the elderly, it was found that the elderly were more likely to manifest less-specific symptoms such as breathlessness, heart failure, dizziness, syncope, neurologic, and psychiatric symptoms. Non-specific symptoms were 2–5 times higher and mortality was approximately 4 times higher (31% versus 7.7%) in those older than 65 [24].

It is very tempting to minimize complaints of dyspnea in the psychiatric population and attribute it to anxiety or exacerbation of existing psychoses. The reality is that true organic disease exists in this population and may even be more prevalent in patients with underlying psychiatric illnesses. Patients with hypoxia and hypercarbia often complain of anxiety and can manifest behavioral changes. Subsequently the complaint of dyspnea in this patient population should be treated as aggressively as in patients without psychiatric illness. Screening with pulse oximetry is essential along with a focused cardiopulmonary examination in search of abnormalities in the anxious or altered patient.

Pitfall | **Not including pulmonary embolism in the differential diagnosis of the patient with dyspnea**

Pulmonary embolism (PE) can frequently be a very difficult disease to diagnose. Its presentation is often subtle and difficult to distinguish from other diseases. This is even more apparent in patients with underlying cardiopulmonary pathology. Perhaps the best quote on PE was provided by Laack et al. "Regardless of the presentation, the most fundamental step in making the diagnosis of PE is first to consider it" [25]. Dyspnea is the most common symptom of PE [26].

The exact incidence and mortality due to PE remains uncertain. Some sources report that the incidence is between 200,000 and 300,000 cases per year [27–29]. The number of deaths has been estimated to range from 50,000 to 100,000 per year [29]. However, when properly diagnosed and treated, clinically apparent pulmonary emboli are an uncommon cause of death [30].

> KEY FACT | Using objective criteria to assess pre-test probability of PE will allow the clinician to cater the workup of the patient to the likelihood of disease, thus avoiding unnecessary tests and ensuring that a PE is not ruled out by using a test that is not sensitive enough for the clinical scenario.

Patients suspected of having a PE should be risk stratified by their pre-test clinical probability of disease. One simple objective prediction rule is the Wells Criteria [31]. Fedullo and Tapson report, "25–65% of patients with suspected embolism are categorized as having a low clinical probability of embolism; in this subgroup, the prevalence of PE ranges from 5% to 10%. Another 25–65% of patients with suspected embolism are categorized as having an intermediate clinical probability of embolism; in this subgroup, the prevalence of PE ranges from 25% to 45%" [32]. Such diagnostic criteria has the potential to reduce morbidity and mortality in cases of thromboembolism by identifying those at varying levels of risk and thus allowing the workup to be adjusted accordingly.

Pitfall | **Over-reliance on the D-dimer, arterial blood gas (ABG), CXR, or EKG to exclude PE**

> KEY FACT | D-dimer assays vary considerably in their sensitivity. It is imperative that clinicians are aware of the characteristics of the assays used in their institutions and that they apply the results on an appropriate patient population.

D-dimer is often used in the ED during the evaluation of PE. However, there are some important limitations to this test. Several different D-dimer assays exist and there is considerable variability in their test characteristics making the generalizability of published estimates of D-dimer accuracy difficult [33]. There are latex agglutination tests and enzyme-linked immunosorbent assay (ELISA) tests. Some latex agglutination tests may only have a sensitivity of 65% and a negative predictive value of 81% [34]. However, a meta-analysis concluded that the ELISAs in general yield better sensitivities (of approximately 95%) [35]. Additionally, there are certain scenarios in which D-dimer tests may be problematic. Patients who have had recent surgery (within 3 months) and patients with cancer may have elevated D-dimer levels making this test non-specific in this patient population. Furthermore, in these high-risk patients, because the pre-test probability is high at baseline, the negative predictive value of the D-dimer test is only 80% [36]. Finally, D-dimer assays may be affected by clot burden and location of the emboli. There is greater accuracy in excluding segmental or larger emboli (sensitivity 93%) than subsegmental emboli (sensitivity = 50%). D-dimer concentration and the accuracy of D-dimer assays are clearly dependent on embolus location and smaller, subsegmental emboli may be missed when D-dimer assays are used as a sole test to exclude PE [37]. Patients with a low pre-test probability of PE are the only ones in whom a D-dimer has any utility to exclude disease. Furthermore, only ultrasensitive D-dimers should be used to exclude venothromboembolism in these patients. Presently, the sensitivity of qualitative and latex agglutination D-dimer assays is not sufficient to exclude disease in even these low-risk patients.

There have been multiple proposed diagnostic algorithims which incorporate clinical assessment, imaging studies (lower extremity ultrasound, V/Q scan, computed tomography (CT) scan), and D-dimer tests. While some advocate the cessation of a workup when there is a low pre-test clinical probability and an ELISA D-dimer <500 ng/ml, none currently advocate the use of a negative D-dimer with a high or intermediate pre-test probability.

ABG data alone or in combination with other clinical data is not useful in the assessment of suspected PE [38]. Patients with acute PE are classically described as having hypoxemia, hypocapnia, an elevated alveolar–arterial oxygen gradient and a respiratory alkalosis. However, not all patients will exhibit these findings. Some patients, particularly the young, may not present with hypoxia or an elevated alveolar–arterial oxygen gradient [39]. Up to 6% of patients with PE will have a normal alveolar–arterial oxygen gradient. [26] In addition, patients with a large PE may actually have hypercapnia and respiratory acidosis secondary to circulatory and ventilatory collapse. The ABG should not be not be used to exclude or establish the diagnosis of PE.

> KEY FACT | **Radiographic findings with PE may mimic those of pneumonia or pleural effusions.**

The chest X-ray (CXR) cannot prove or exclude PE. A normal chest radiograph in the setting of severe dyspnea and hypoxemia without other cardiopulmonary findings is strongly suggestive of PE [40]. However, the majority of patients with PE will have an abnormal chest radiograph. Common findings include atelectasis, pulmonary infiltrates, pleural effusion, and elevated hemidiaphragm. Classically taught findings such as Hampton's hump or decreased vascularity (Westermark's sign) are suggestive but uncommon [26, 40, 41]. Findings of pulmonary infarction can sometimes be mistaken for infiltrates, thereby causing clinicians to mistakenly diagnose patients with pneumonia. In addition, the presence of a pleural effusion increases the likelihood of PE in young patients who present with acute pleuritic chest pain [42]. This again highlights the importance of considering the diagnosis of PE. If it is not in the differential diagnosis, the possibility of PE will not be entertained.

The classic electrocardiographic findings with PE have been described as the traditional S1Q3T3 pattern characterized by a large S-wave in lead I, and a Q-wave and T-wave inversion in lead III. While often considered the hallmark of PE, these findings are neither sensitive nor specific for PE. Though sinus tachycardia is the most frequently encountered rhythm, normal EKGs are encountered in approximately 10–25% of patients with PE [43]. Patterns indicative of right ventricular strain are also suggestive of PE [44].

> Electrocardiographic findings of right ventricular strain suggestive of PE [44].
>
> - Incomplete or complete right bundle branch block
> - Large S-waves in leads I and aVL
> - Shift in transition zone in the precordial leads to V5
> - Q-waves in leads III and aVF
> - Right axis deviation
> - Low-voltage QRS in limb leads
> - T-wave inversion in inferior and anterior leads

Pitfall | **Relying on a normal CXR to rule out cardiopulmonary disease**

> KEY FACT | **In patients with unexplained dyspnea and normal findings on routine studies, clinicians should have a heightened suspicion for PE and myocardial or pericardial disease.**

The seasoned clinician should immediately recognize that a normal CXR does very little to help one exclude many cardiopulmonary causes of dyspnea. With the exception of tension pneumothorax, most life-threatening causes of dyspnea may demonstrate a normal CXR. Included in this partial list are airway obstruction, PE, myocardial infarction, congestive heart failure, cardiac tamponade, asthma, cor pulmonale, pneumonia, pericarditis, COPD exacerbation, pulmonary hypertension, myocarditis, carbon monoxide poisoning, and methemoglobinemia. Small pneumothoracies may also be missed in recumbent patients, especially when the pneumothorax is located anteriorly. In addition, if the CXR is an anteroposterior (AP) or portable view, the sensitivity is perhaps even lower. The negative predictive value of a chest radiograph is not sufficient to exclude cardiopulmonary disease. In a case where a CXR is read as normal in a hypoxic and dyspneic patient, the likelihood of cardiac and thromboembolic pathology increases. This warrants the further investigation of venothromboembolism and pericardial/ myocardial disease states with the consideration of bedside echocardiography, EKG, cardiac enzymes, and possibly chest CT. In fact, in one ED study, of 103 patients with unexplained dyspnea who then underwent bedside echocardiography, 14 (13.6%) had pericardial effusions [45]. Of these four were felt to be large enough to explain the patients' dyspnea.

Pitfall | Overly or underly aggressive oxygen administration in patients with COPD

The traditional teaching has been that administration of oxygen will cause the spontaneously breathing COPD patient in respiratory distress to "stop breathing." It was traditionally taught that suppression of the hypoxic ventilatory drive would lead to hypercapnia and subsequent hypercapnic respiratory failure. However, it appears as though our traditional understanding of the pathophysiology was incorrect. Three mechanisms have been shown to worsen hypercapnia when oxygen is administered in the COPD patient:

1. Worsened V/Q matching due to a decrease in hypoxic pulmonary vasoconstriction (HPV);
2. Decreased binding affinity of hemoglobin for CO_2;
3. Decreased minute ventilation [46, 47].

HPV is a physiologic response to alveolar hypoxia. Through this mechanism blood is diverted away from poorly ventilated lung units. When hypoxia affects the entire lung (typically occurs at PaO_2 levels <60 mmHg), HPV occurs throughout the lung. This increases the pulmonary artery pressure and subsequently recruits many previously unperfused pulmonary capillaries, increasing the surface area available for gas diffusion, and improving the matching of ventilation and perfusion. If the hypoxia is resolved with supplemental oxygen, HPV is blunted, thus worsening V/Q matching. This essentially increases the physiologic deadspace and shunt and subsequently leads to elevations in PCO_2 [46, 48].

The CO_2 dissociation curve shifts to the right in the presence of increased oxygen saturation. This is known as the Haldane effect. Subsequently, in the presence of increased oxygen saturation from supplemental oxygen, oxyhemoglobin binds CO_2 less avidly than deoxyhemoglobin, thus increasing the amount of CO_2 dissolved in blood. This in turn is reflected as an increased $PaCO_2$ [49].

Administration of supplemental oxygen to a COPD patient in respiratory distress has also been show to decrease the patient's minute ventilation. This is due to a small decrease in respiratory rate that will also increase PCO_2 [47].

As a general rule, prevention of tissue hypoxia is more important than CO_2 retention concerns. Many patients with COPD have a chronic compensated respiratory acidosis. While normal individuals may begin to experience depressed level of consciousness at $PaCO_2$ levels of 60–70 mmHg, COPD patients may not exhibit these symptoms until their $PaCO_2$ reaches a level in excess of 90–100 mmHg. COPD patients are at greater risk from hypoxia than from hypercapnia and oxygen should not be withheld from the hypoxic COPD patient. Oxygen therapy should be emergently initiated in all hypoxic COPD patients with an initial goal oxygen saturation of 88–92% unless there is evidence of active cardiac or cerebral ischemia.

The primary goal of oxygen therapy is to prevent tissue hypoxia. The American Thoracic Society/European Respiratory Society recommends a SaO_2 greater than 90% or a PaO_2 of 60–70 mmHg [50]. In addition, Kelly et al. reported that oxygen saturation by pulse oximetry may be an effective screening test for systemic hypoxia, with the screening cutoff of 92% having sensitivity for the detection of systemic hypoxia of 100% with specificity of 86% [51]. Further increases in the FiO_2 above the level needed to achieve these goals do not add significantly to the oxygen content of blood, but do increase the potential for more severe secondary hypercapnia [50]. Venturi masks should be used when possible to permit tight regulation of FiO_2.

Finally, if CO_2 retention occurs, monitor for acidemia. If acidemia occurs, consider a trial of non-invasive or invasive mechanical ventilation [50].

Pitfall | Not considering non-invasive positive pressure ventilation; that is, CPAP/BiPAP as an alternative to intubation in selected patients

Non-invasive positive pressure ventilation (NPPV) has been shown to reduce length of hospital stay, morbidity, mortality, and need for invasive mechanical ventilation. The data supporting the use of NPPV is strongest for COPD exacerbations; however, there is growing evidence to support its use in cardiogenic pulmonary edema [52–55], hypoxic respiratory failure [56–60], pneumonia [56, 61], immunocompromised states [62, 63], and asthma [64, 65].

There is a wealth of information showing the benefit of NPPV in acute exacerbations of COPD. This data includes randomized controlled trials, systemic reviews, and meta-analysis [66–74]. NPPV has been shown to decrease intubation rates (RR 0.42, 95% CI 0.31–0.59), decrease mortality (RR 0.41, 95% CI 0.26–0.64), decrease complications (RR 0.32, 95% CI 0.18–0.56), and decrease hospital length of stay (weight mean difference −3.24 days, 95% CI −4.42 to −2.26) [68].

It is important to note that early institution of NPPV is vital. Conti et al. showed that if one waits for failure of conventional medical therapy, the benefits conferred by NPPV (length of ICU stay, number of days on mechanical ventilation, overall complications, ICU mortality, and hospital mortality) are eliminated [75]. As such, patients in respiratory distress, not requiring emergent intubation and without contraindications should be considered for NPPV. The American Association for Respiratory Care recommends the early use of NPPV when two or more of the following are present:

1. Respiratory distress with moderate to severe dyspnea.
2. Arterial pH <7.35 with $PaCO_2$ above 45 mmHg.
3. Respiratory rate of ≥ 25/min [76].

Improvement should be seen within 30–60 min, and if improvement does not occur within 1–2 h, invasive mechanical ventilation should be initiated. One should also be aware that when using NPPV, frequent checks and adjustments are required. Failure to do so may lead to the patient's condition worsening and a delay in the institution of invasive mechanical ventilation.

Pearls for Improving Patient Outcomes

- Do not rely solely on a normal physical examination to exclude disease.
- Patients with a normal pulse oximetry may still suffer from ventilatory failure.
- Shortness of breath should be attributed to anxiety only when all other causes have been definitively excluded.
- Risk stratification of patients with suspected venous thromboembolism utilizing clinical decision rules will aid in the diagnosis of PE.
- A normal CXR does very little to exclude cardiopulmonary causes of dyspnea.
- The negative predictive value of a normal ABG or CXR does not allow one to exclude PE.
- A D-dimer test should not be used to exclude PE in patients with moderate or high clinic pre-test probability.
- Only high-sensitivity D-Dimer tests should be used to exclude PE in patients but should only be used in patients with a low pre-test probability.
- Do not withhold oxygen from a hypoxic COPD patient; however, be cautious with its use and follow PCO_2 levels.
- Consider the use of NPPV in selected patients with respiratory distress if they do not require immediate emergent intubation. This is especially true with patients in COPD exacerbation.

References

1. Dyspnea. Mechanisms, assessment, and management: a consensus statement. American Thoracic Society. *Am J Respir Crit Care Med* 1999; 159:321.
2. Banzett RB, Mulnier HE, Murphy K, Rosen SD, Wise RJ, Adams L. Breathlessness in humans activates insular cortex. *NeuroReport* 2000; 11(10):2117–20.
3. O'Connor GT, Anderson KM, Kannel WB, et al. Prevalence and prognosis of dyspnea in the Farmingham Study. *Chest* 1987; 92:90S.
4. Hirshberg A, Thomson SR, Huizinga WK. Reliability of physical examination in penetrating chest injuries. *Injury* 1988; 19(6): 407–9.
5. Chen SC, Chang KJ, Hsu CY. Accuracy of auscultation in the detection of haemopneumothorax. *Eur J Surg* 1998; 164(9):643–5.
6. Chen SC, Markmann JF, Kauder DR, Schwab CW. Hemopneumothorax missed by auscultation in penetrating chest injury. *J Trauma* 1997; 42(1):86–89.
7. Bokhari F, Brakenridge S, Nagy K, Roberts R, Smith R, Joseph K, An G, Wiley D, Barrett J. Prospective evaluation of the sensitivity of physical examination in chest trauma. *J Trauma* 2002; 53(6):1135–8.
8. Wipf JE, Lipsky BA, Hirschmann JV, Boyko EJ, Takasugi J, Peugeot RL, Davis CL. Diagnosing pneumonia by physical examination: relevant or relic? *Arch Intern Med* 1999; 159 (10): 1082–7.
9. Metlay JP, Kapoor WN, Fine MJ. Does this patient have community-acquired pneumonia? Diagnosing pneumonia by history and physical examination. *J Am Med Assoc* 1997; 278(17):1440–5.
10. Chakko S, Woska D, Martinez H, et al. Clinical, radiographic, and hemodynamic correlations in chronic congestive heart failure: conflicting results may lead to inappropriate care. *Am J Med* 1991; 90:353–9.
11. Witting MD, Hsu S, Granja CA. The sensitivity of room-air pulse oximetry in the detection of hypercapnia. *Am J Emerg Med* 2005; 23(4):497–500.
12. Witting MD, Lueck CH. The ability of pulse oximetry to screen for hypoxemia and hypercapnia in patients breathing room air. *J Emerg Med* 2001; 20(4):341–8.
13. Ayas N, Bergstrom LR, Schwab TR, Narr BJ. Unrecognized severe postoperative hypercapnia: a case of apneic oxygenation. *Mayo Clin Proc* 1998; 73(1):51–54.
14. Potkin RT, Swenson ER. Resuscitation from severe acute hypercapnia. Determinants of tolerance and survival. *Chest* 1992; 102(6):1742–5.
15. Stoneham MD. Uses and limitations of pulse oximetry. *Br J Hosp Med* 1995; 54(1):35–41.
16. Hampson NB. Pulse oximetry in severe carbon monoxide poisoning. *Chest* 1998; 114(4):1036–41.
17. Miner JR, Heegaard W, Plummer D. End-tidal carbon dioxide monitoring during procedural sedation. *Acad Emerg Med* 2002; 9(4):275–80.
18. Rohling R, Biro P. Clinical investigation of a new combined pulse oximetry and carbon dioxide tension sensor in adult anaesthesia. *J Clin Monit Comput* 1999; 15(1):23–27.
19. Senn O, Clarenbach CF, Kaplan V, Maggiorini M, Bloch KE. Monitoring carbon dioxide tension and arterial oxygen saturation by a single earlobe sensor in patients with critical illness or sleep apnea. *Chest* 2005; 128(3):1291–6.
20. Chhajed PN, Kaegi B, Rajasekaran R, Tamm M. Detection of hypoventilation during thoracoscopy: combined cutaneous carbon dioxide tension and oximetry monitoring with a new digital sensor. *Chest* 2005; 127(2):585–8.
21. Yohannes AM, Roomi J, Baldwin RC, Connolly MJ. Depression in elderly outpatients with disabling chronic obstructive pulmonary disease. *Age Ageing* 1998; 27(2):155–60.
22. Horton-Deutsch SL, Clark DC, Farran CJ. Chronic dyspnea and suicide in elderly men. *Hosp Commun Psychiatr* 1992; 43(12): 1198–203.

23. Ben-Dov I. Fatal asthma: who, when, why and how to prevent? *Harefuah* 2002; 141(6):524–6, 579, 578.

24. de Fockert JA. Clinical presentation of acute myocardial infarct in the elderly. *Tijdschr Gerontol Geriatr* 1987; 18(6):305–8.

25. Laack TA, Goyal DG. Pulmonary embolism: an unsuspected killer. *Emerg Med Clin N Am* 2004; 22(4):961–83.

26. Stein, PD, Terrin, ML, Hales, CA, et al. Clinical, laboratory, roentgenographic, and electrocardiographic findings in patients with acute pulmonary embolism and no pre-existing cardiac or pulmonary disease. *Chest* 1991; 100:598.

27. Anderson Jr FA, Wheeler HB, Goldberg RJ, et al. A population-based perspective of the hospital incidence and case-fatality rates of deep vein thrombosis and pulmonary embolism: the Worcester DVT Study. *Arch Intern Med* 1991; 151:933–8.

28. Silverstein MD, Heit JA, Mohr DN, Petterson TM, O'Fallon WM, Melton III LJ. Trends in the incidence of deep vein thrombosis and pulmonary embolism: a 25-year population-based study. *Arch Intern Med* 1998; 158:585–93.

29. Goldhaber SZ. Pulmonary embolism. *New Engl J Med* 1998; 339:93–104.

30. Carson JL, Kelley MA, Duff A, et al. The clinical course of pulmonary embolism. *New Engl J Med* 1992; 326:1240–5.

31. Wolf SJ, McCubbin TR, Feldhaus KM, Faragher JP, Adcock DM. Prospective validation of wells criteria in the evaluation of patients with suspected pulmonary embolism. *Ann Emerg Med* 2004; 44(5):503–10.

32. Fedullo PF, Tapson VF. The evaluation of suspected pulmonary embolism. *New Engl J Med* 2003; 349:1247–56.

33. Becker DM, Philbrick JT, Bachhuber TL, Humphries JE. D-dimer testing and acute venous thromboembolism. A shortcut to accurate diagnosis? *Arch Intern Med* 1996; 156(9):939–46.

34. Farrell S, Hayes T, Shaw M. A negative SimpliRED D-dimer assay result does not exclude the diagnosis of deep vein thrombosis or pulmonary embolus in emergency department patients. *Ann Emerg Med* 2000; 35(2):121–5.

35. Stein PD, Hull RD, Patel KC, Olson RE, Ghali WA, Brant R, Biel RK, Bharadia V, Kalra NK. D-dimer for the exclusion of acute venous thrombosis and pulmonary embolism: a systematic review. *Ann Intern Med* 2004; 140(8):589–602.

36. Lee AY, Julian JA, Levine MN, Weitz JI, Kearon C, Wells PS, Ginsberg JS. Clinical utility of a rapid whole-blood D-dimer assay in patients with cancer who present with suspected acute deep venous thrombosis. *Ann Intern Med* 1999; 131(6):417–23.

37. De Monye W, Sanson BJ, Mac Gillavry MR, Pattynama PM, Buller HR, van den Berg-Huysmans AA, Huisman MV. Embolus location affects the sensitivity of a rapid quantitative D-dimer assay in the diagnosis of pulmonary embolism. *Am J Respir Crit Care Med* 2002; 165(3):345–8.

38. Rodger MA, Carrier M, Jones GN, Rasuli P, Raymond F, Djunaedi H, Wells PS. Diagnostic value of arterial blood gas measurement in suspected pulmonary embolism. *Am J Respir Crit Care Med* 2000; 162(6):2105–8.

39. Green RM, Meyer TJ, Dunn M, Glassroth J. Pulmonary embolism in younger adults. *Chest* 1992; 101(6):1507–11.

40. ATS guidelines: the diagnostic approach to acute venous thromboembolism. *Am J Respir Crit Care Med* 1999; 160:1043.

41. Worsley DF, Alavi A, Aronchick JM, Chen JT, Greenspan RH, Ravin CE. Chest radiographic findings in patients with acute pulmonary embolism: observations from the PIOPED study. *Radiology* 1993; 189(1):133–6.

42. McNeill BJ, Hessel SJ, Branch WT, et al. Measures of clinical efficacy: 3. The value of the lung scan in the evaluation of young patients with pleuritic chest pain. *J Nucl Med* 1976; 17:163.

43. Ullman E, Brady WJ, Perron AD, Chan T, Mattu A. Electrocardiographic manifestations of pulmonary embolism. *Am J Emerg Med* 2001; 19:514–9.

44. Sreeram N, Cheriex EC, Smeets JLRM, et al. Value of the 12-lead electrocardiogram at hospital admission in the diagnosis of pulmonary embolism. *Am J Cardiol* 1994; 73:298–303.

45. Blaivas M. Incidence of pericardial effusion in patients presenting to the emergency department with unexplained dyspnea. *Acad Emerg Med* 2001; 8(12):1143–6.

46. Aubier M, Murciano D, Milic-Emili J, Touaty E, Daghfous J, Pariente R, Derenne JP. Effects of the administration of O_2 on ventilation and blood gases in patients with chronic obstructive pulmonary disease during acute respiratory failure. *Am Rev Respir Dis* 1980; 122(5):747–54.

47. Aubier M, Murciano D, Fournier M, Milic-Emili J, Pariente R, Derenne JP. Central respiratory drive in acute respiratory failure of patients with chronic obstructive pulmonary disease. *Am Rev Respir Dis* 1980; 122(2):191–9.

48. Levitzky MG. *Pulmonary Physiology*, 6th edn. New York: McGraw-Hill/Appleton & Lange, 2003, p. 107.

49. Levitzky MG. *Pulmonary Physiology*, 6th edn. New York: McGraw-Hill/Appleton & Lange, 2003, pp. 158–9.

50. Standards for the diagnosis and care of patients with chronic obstructive pulmonary disease. American Thoracic Society. *Am J Respir Crit Care Med* 1995; 152:S77.

51. Kelly AM, McAlpine R, Kyle E. *Respir Med* 2001; 95(5):336–40.

52. Wigder HN, Hoffman P, Mazzolini D, et al. Pressure support noninvasive positive pressure ventilation treatment of acute cardiogenic pulmonary edema. *Am J Emerg Med* 2001; 19: 179–81.

53. Pang D, Keenan S, Cook D, et al. The effect of positive pressure airway support on mortality and the need for intubation in cardiogenic pulmonary edema. A systematic review. *Chest* 1998; 114(4):1185–92.

54. Bersten AD, Holt AW, Vedig AE, Skowronski GA, Baggoley CJ. Treatment of severe cardiogenic pulmonary edema with continuous positive airway pressure delivered by face mask. *New Engl J Med* 1991; 325(26):1825–30.

55. Nava S, Carbone G, DiBattista N, Bellone A, Baiardi P, Cosentini R, Marenco M, Giostra F, Borasi G, Groff P. Noninvasive ventilation in cardiogenic pulmonary edema: a multicenter randomized trial. *Am J Respir Crit Care Med* 2003; 168(12):1432–7.

56. Ferrer M, Esquinas A, Leon M, Gonzalez G, Alarcon A, Torres A. Noninvasive ventilation in severe hypoxemic respiratory failure: a randomized clinical trial. *Am J Respir Crit Care Med* 2003; 168(12):1438–44.

57. Antonelli M, Conti G, Rocco M, Bufi M, De Blasi RA, Vivino G, Gasparetto A, Meduri GU. A comparison of noninvasive positive-pressure ventilation and conventional mechanical ventilation in patients with acute respiratory failure. *New Engl J Med* 1998; 339(7):429–35.

58. Martin TJ, Hovis JD, Costantino JP, Bierman MI, Donahoe MP, Rogers RM, Kreit JW, Sciurba FC, Stiller RA, Sanders MH. A randomized, prospective evaluation of noninvasive ventilation for acute respiratory failure. *Am J Respir Crit Care Med* 2000; 161(3 Pt 1):807–13.

59. Delclaux C, L'Her E, Alberti C, Mancebo J, Abroug F, Conti G, Guerin C, Schortgen F, Lefort Y, Antonelli M, Lepage E, Lemaire F, Brochard L. Treatment of acute hypoxemic nonhypercapnic respiratory insufficiency with continuous positive airway pressure delivered by a face mask: a randomized controlled trial. *J Am Med Assoc* 2000; 284(18):2352–60.

60. Keenan SP, Sinuff T, Cook DJ, Hill NS. Does noninvasive positive pressure ventilation improve outcome in acute hypoxemic respiratory failure? A systematic review. *Crit Care Med* 2004; 32(12):2516–23.

61. Confalonieri M, Potena A, Carbone G, Porta RD, Tolley EA, Umberto Meduri G. Acute respiratory failure in patients with severe community-acquired pneumonia. A prospective randomized evaluation of noninvasive ventilation. *Am J Respir Crit Care Med* 1999; 160(5 Pt 1):1585–91.

62. Confalonieri M, Calderini E, Terraciano S, Chidini G, Celeste E, Puccio G, Gregoretti C, Meduri GU. Noninvasive ventilation for treating acute respiratory failure in AIDS patients with Pneumocystis carinii pneumonia. *Intens Care Med* 2002; 28(9):1233–8.

63. Hilbert G, Gruson D, Vargas F, Valentino R, Gbikpi-Benissan G, Dupon M, Reiffers J, Cardinaud JP. Noninvasive ventilation in immunosuppressed patients with pulmonary infiltrates, fever, and acute respiratory failure. *New Engl J Med* 2001; 344(7):481–7.

64. Soroksky A, Stav D, Shpirer I. A pilot prospective, randomized, placebo-controlled trial of bilevel positive airway pressure in acute asthmatic attack. *Chest* 2003; 123(4):1018–25.

65. Meduri GU, Cook TR, Turner RE, et al. Noninvasive positive pressure ventilation in status asthmaticus. *Chest* 1996; 110(3):767–74.

66. Brochard L, Mancebo J, Wysocki M, Lofaso F, Conti G, Rauss A, Simonneau G, Benito S, Gasparetto A, Lemaire F. Noninvasive ventilation for acute exacerbations of chronic obstructive pulmonary disease. *New Engl J Med* 1995; 333(13):817–22.

67. Wysocki M, Tric L, Wolff MA, Millet H, Herman B. Noninvasive pressure support ventilation in patients with acute respiratory failure. A randomized comparison with conventional therapy. *Chest* 1995; 107(3):761–8.

68. Ram FS, Picot J, Lightowler J, Wedzicha JA. Non-invasive positive pressure ventilation for treatment of respiratory failure due to exacerbations of chronic obstructive pulmonary disease. *Cochrane Database Syst Rev* 2004; (3):CD004104.

69. Peter JV, Moran JL, Phillips-Hughes J, Warn D. Noninvasive ventilation in acute respiratory failure—a meta-analysis update. *Crit Care Med* 2002; 30(3):555–62.

70. Lightowler JV, Wedzicha JA, Elliott MW, Ram FS. Non-invasive positive pressure ventilation to treat respiratory failure resulting from exacerbations of chronic obstructive pulmonary disease: cochrane systematic review and meta-analysis. *Br Med J* 2003; 326(7382):185.

71. Keenan SP, Sinuff T, Cook DJ, Hill NS. Which patients with acute exacerbation of chronic obstructive pulmonary disease benefit from noninvasive positive-pressure ventilation? A systematic review of the literature. *Ann Intern Med* 2003; 138(11):861–70.

72. Plant PK, Owen JL, Elliott MW. Early use of noninvasive ventilation for acute exacerbations of chronic obstructive pulmonary disease on general respiratory wards: a multicentre randomised controlled trial. *Lancet* 2000; 355:1931–5.

73. Keenan SP, Gregor J, Sibbald WJ, et al. Noninvasive positive pressure ventilation in the setting of severe, acute exacerbations of chronic obstructive pulmonary disease: more effective and less expensive. *Crit Care Med* 2000; 28(6):2094–103.

74. Celikel T, Sungur M, Ceyhan B, et al. Comparisons of noninvasive positive pressure ventilation with standard medical therapy in acute hypercapneic respiratory failure. *Chest* 1998; 114(6):1636–42.

75. Conti G, Antonelli M, Navalesi P, et al. Noninvasive vs. conventional mechanical ventilation in patients with chronic obstructive pulmonary disease after failure of medical treatment in the ward: a randomized trial. *Intens Care Med* 2002; 28(12):1701–7.

76. Bach, JR, Brougher, P, Hess, DR, et al. Consensus conference: noninvasive positive pressure ventilation. *Respir Care* 1997; 42:364–9.

Chapter 3 | Evaluation and Management of the Patient with Abdominal Pain

Joseph P. Martinez

Introduction

Abdominal pain is the most commonly cited reason for a visit to an emergency department (ED), accounting for nearly 7% of all ED encounters [1]. A great majority of patients will be discharged; many with the diagnosis of undifferentiated abdominal pain (UDAP). Approximately 10% of these patients will require urgent or emergent surgery [2]. The evaluation of the patient with abdominal pain is fraught with hazards ranging from the subjectivity of the pain itself, to the myriad of diagnostic possibilities. Serious pathology can affect patients of all ages, from the newborn with malrotation to the geriatric patient with intestinal ischemia. The astute clinician must be able to distinguish between those patients that can safely be discharged home, those patients that need further evaluation in the ED or inpatient setting, and those that require emergent intervention to ward off impending mortality.

Pitfall | Misdiagnosis of cardiac ischemia as intra-abdominal pathology (and vice versa)

> KEY FACT | [Of] elderly patients presenting with unstable angina … 45% had no chest pain. Eight percent … presented with epigastric pain.

Pathology on one side of the diaphragm can cause symptoms on the opposite side. The most crucial example of this is acute coronary syndrome (ACS) masquerading as an intra-abdominal process. It has long been recognized that a large percentage of patients with ACS will present without chest pain. Atypical presentations are more common in women, diabetics, and elderly patients [3, 4]. Canto et al. examined elderly patients presenting with unstable angina and found that 45% had no chest pain; 8% of patients presented with epigastric pain, 38% with nausea, and 11% with vomiting [5]. A review of the data from the National Registry of Myocardial Infarction-2 again showed that one-third of patients had no chest pain. Upper abdominal pain was often instead the presenting complaint. Patients presenting without chest pain were on average 7 years older, more likely to be women, and a significantly higher number

were diabetics. Patients that presented atypically experienced longer delays and underwent reperfusion less often. They were also less likely to receive medications such as aspirin, heparin, or beta-blockers. Most importantly, they had a mortality rate of 23% as opposed to 9% in the typical group [3]. This data underscores the importance of considering cardiac ischemia in patients presenting with gastrointestinal complaints. In patients at risk for cardiac disease, an electrocardiogram should be obtained just as urgently as if the patient were presenting with chest pain.

Conversely, it is well-reported in the literature that some intra-abdominal conditions can mimic myocardial infarction, most notably pancreatitis, but also acute cholecystitis (AC). The literature is replete with cases of acute pancreatitis (AP) in which an electrocardiogram shows changes of myocardial ischemia, including ST-segment elevation [6–9]. In several of these cases, the patients have been mistakenly administered thrombolytics [10, 11]. While patients with ACS may complain of abdominal pain, it is unusual for there to be objective abdominal tenderness. If the diagnosis is unclear, consideration should be made to further evaluate the patient with serial electrocardiograms or emergent coronary angiography. Thrombolytic therapy should be withheld if there is any concern that the patient's symptoms may actually represent pancreatitis, peptic ulcer disease (PUD), or aortic dissection.

Pitfall | Over-reliance on laboratory values and ancillary testing in suspected mesenteric ischemia

The incidence of mesenteric ischemia is low, approximately 1 in 1000 hospital admissions; however, it accounts for 1 out of every 100 admissions for abdominal pain [12]. Clearly, most emergency physicians (EPs) are seeing patients with mesenteric ischemia, whether or not they recognize it. The diagnosis of mesenteric ischemia should be entertained in every patient with a complaint of severe abdominal pain and a paucity of physical findings (the classic "pain out of proportion to exam"). Elucidation of risk factors can also suggest the diagnosis (see Table 3.1). Acute superior mesenteric artery (SMA) embolus is more common in patients with underlying cardiac disease. The most common cardiac conditions that predispose

Table 3.1 Risk factors for mesenteric ischemia.

Type of mesenteric ischemia	Risk factors	Special notes
SMA embolus	Cardiac disease • Atrial fibrillation or other arrhythmia • Valvular disease • Ventricular aneurysm • Cardiomyopathy	One-third have a history of a previous embolic event
SMA thrombosis	Vascular disease risks • Hypertension • Hypercholesterolemia • Diabetes mellitus • Smoking	Acute event may be preceded by period of "intestinal angina" and prolonged period of significant weight loss
Mesenteric venous thrombosis	Hypercoaguable state • Inherited (factor V Leiden mutation, etc.) • Acquired (malignancy, oral contraceptives, etc.)	One-half have personal or family history of DVT/PE Subacute presentation Women > men
NOMI	Low-flow states • Sepsis • Heart failure • Volume depletion Hemodialysis Drugs • Digitalis • Ergot derivatives • Cocaine • Norepinephrine Post-surgery	Often ICU patients

DVT: deep venous thrombosis; PE: pulmonary embolus; NOMI: non-occlusive mesenteric ischemia; ICU: intensive care unit.

to SMA embolus are atrial fibrillation, other arrhythmias, previous myocardial infarction with ventricular aneurysm formation, valvular heart disease, or dilated cardiomyopathy [13]. Physical findings of previous embolic disease such as prior stroke or amputated toes may increase suspicion. SMA thrombosis is seen in patients with classic cardiovascular risk factors. These patients should be specifically interrogated for symptoms of previous "intestinal ischemia" – abdominal pain provoked by meals. They may also demonstrate significant unintentional weight loss. One-half of patients with mesenteric venous thrombosis will have a personal or family history of deep venous thrombosis or pulmonary embolus [14]. They should be interviewed as would any patient in whom you suspect a thromboembolic process. Close attention should be paid to clues that suggest inherited thrombophilias – family history of thromboembolic events, multiple first trimester pregnancy losses, or previous personal clot history. Acquired risks such as smoking or oral contraceptive use should also be investigated. Non-occlusive mesenteric ischemia should be near the top of the differential diagnosis list in any patient that exhibits a "low-flow state" and presents with abdominal pain. This would include patients that are septic, severely volume depleted, or with

end-stage congestive heart failure, and those that use cocaine, digitalis, or are on hemodialysis [15–17].

> KEY FACT | **Mortality from mesenteric ischemia is nearly 80% ... With immediate angiography, the mortality rate could be reduced to 54%.**

Mortality from mesenteric ischemia is nearly 80%. This mortality rate has remained remarkably constant through the years. A landmark study by Boley et al. finally demonstrated improvement in mortality only through the aggressive use of early angiography. His group showed that with immediate angiography, the mortality rate could be reduced to 54% [18]. These results have since been duplicated in a number of other studies [19, 20]. Unfortunately, many physicians are unwilling to obtain angiography based solely on the patient's presentation and risk factors. They will wait for collateral laboratory data, and obtain other, suboptimal imaging. This is akin to delaying reperfusion in ACS until the cardiac enzymes have peaked. While an elevated lactate level, leukocytosis, metabolic acidosis, and hyperamylasemia support the diagnosis, none of them are sensitive enough to rule it out completely. In addition, obtaining other imaging studies merely delays the time required to obtain a definitive angiographic diagnosis and start treatment. If the patient has risk factors for mesenteric ischemia, and the history and physical examination suggest this diagnosis, arrangements should be made for immediate angiography and surgical consultation. The following caveats apply: (1) If mesenteric venous thrombosis is suspected, computed tomography (CT) is better than angiography [21], unless the angiographer is specifically instructed to perform venous phase angiography. (2) If there will be a long delay in obtaining angiography and the ED has access to a multi-detector row CT scanner, a "mesenteric ischemia protocol," and interpretation of the images in a timely fashion, CT-angiography shows a great deal of promise as a screening modality (see Figure 3.1) [22].

Pitfall | Failure to consider heterotopic pregnancy in women receiving reproductive assistance

Women of child-bearing age are another high-risk demographic group when presenting with abdominal pain. Most EPs are well versed in the need to evaluate these patients for possible ectopic pregnancy should they present while early in pregnancy. The standard practice for ruling out an ectopic pregnancy is to obtain an ultrasound, transabdominal or endovaginal depending on their gestational age at presentation and/or quantitative ß-HCG count. The diagnosis of ectopic pregnancy is considered "ruled out" if an intrauterine pregnancy (IUP) with fetal heart rate is visualized [23]. In general practice, this is a reasonable approach: heterotopic pregnancy (simultaneous occurrence of two or more implantation sites, usually intrauterine and ectopic) is a rare event, with most estimates in the range of 1:30,000 pregnancies [24].

> **KEY FACT** | **Women receiving ART have rates of heterotopic pregnancy as high as 1:100 pregnancies.**

With the advent of assisted reproductive technology (ART), this ratio has changed. Women receiving ART have rates of heterotopic pregnancy as high as 1:100 pregnancies [25]. This appears to be independent of whether the patient received an ovulation-inducing agent (e.g., clomiphene), an exogenous gonadotropin, or in vitro fertilization with embryo transfer [26–28]. Heterotopic pregnancy in natural conception cycles is rare, though the incidence appears to be increasing [29].

Diagnosing a heterotopic pregnancy requires an extremely high index of suspicion. Women have often already been diagnosed with an IUP by ultrasound. The level of ß-HCG may be increasing appropriately due to the presence of a

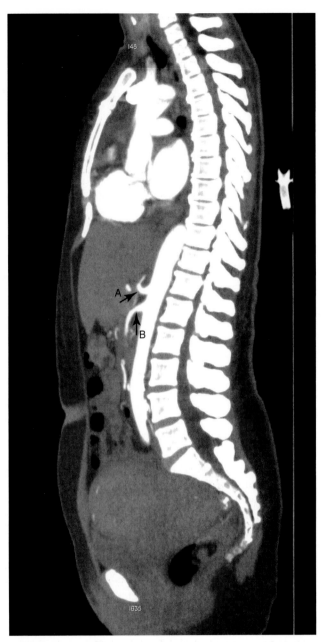

Figure 3.1 Normal mesenteric CT angiogram.
Sagittal reformatting of multi-detector row CT scan (CT angiography) demonstrating normal celiac axis (arrow A) and normal SMA (arrow B).

normal IUP. Adnexal masses and free fluid in the cul-de-sac may be mistakenly attributed to ruptured corpus luteum cysts, an admittedly more common diagnosis. In fact, only 10% of heterotopic gestations are diagnosed prior to operative intervention [25].

A retrospective review of 66 cases of heterotopic pregnancy elucidated 4 common signs and symptoms to help suggest the diagnosis: (1) abdominal pain, (2) adnexal mass, (3) peritoneal irritation, and (4) enlarged uterus [24]. If the diagnosis is made in the first trimester, an enlarged uterus may be absent. More recently, it has been demonstrated that patients with an abnormal amount of free fluid in the cul-de-sac on ultrasound were five times as likely to have an ectopic pregnancy [30]. This finding should not be discounted in any patient, even if a viable IUP is seen. Other findings that should raise a red flag for clinicians include abnormalities seen in the adnexa on ultrasound, especially an echogenic ring surrounding a cystic structure, and relative bradycardia in the face of hemorrhagic shock [31, 32].

Findings suspicious for heterotopic pregnancy.

- Relative bradycardia in the face of hypotension
- Free fluid in cul-de-sac, despite normal IUP
- Adnexal abnormality, especially echogenic ring surrounding cystic structure
- Abdominal pain or peritoneal irritation unexplained by IUP

Pitfall | Over-reliance on "classic" presentations and laboratory results in populations at high risk for atypical presentations of appendicitis

Appendicitis is a common surgical emergency in the general population with a lifetime risk of 7% [33]. Perforation rates range from 17% to 20% [34]. Once thought to be a disease of the young, it is now recognized that 10% of all cases of appendicitis occur in patients over the age of 60 years. While the overall mortality from appendicitis is less than 1%, in the elderly population it ranges from 4% to 8%. This likely reflects the fact that the incidence of perforation in elderly patients is as high as 70% [35].

Dr. Alfredo Alvarado established a practical score known as MANTRELS to assist with the early diagnosis of appendicitis (see Table 3.2). The score is based on typical signs, symptoms, and laboratory values often seen in acute appendicitis, namely: *M*igration of pain, *A*norexia (or ketonuria), *N*ausea and vomiting, *T*enderness in the right lower quadrant, *R*ebound tenderness, *E*levated temperature (>100.4°F, >38°C), *L*eukocytosis (white blood cell (WBC) count >10,400 cells/ml), and *S*hift to

the left (>75% neutrophils). A point is assigned to each, with right lower quadrant tenderness and leukocytosis receiving 2 points, for a total of 10 possible points. A score of 5 or 6 indicates possible appendicitis, 7 or 8 probable appendicitis, and 9 or 10 is very probable appendicitis [36]. This scoring system has been found to be useful as a diagnostic tool in assisting clinicians. Depending on the practice setting, especially when abdominal CT is not readily available for diagnostic purposes, the score can be used to risk stratify patients for discharge with early follow-up, observation, or emergent consultation. If the MANTRELS score is used, it should be weighed in conjunction with physician judgement and should not be used as a means to definitively rule out the possibility of acute appendicitis. Whether or not physicians formally utilize the MANTRELS score, the findings that encompass it are thought to be highly representative of appendicitis.

KEY FACT | **Only 20% of elderly patients will have the classic findings of fever, anorexia, right lower quadrant pain, and leukocytosis.**

Unfortunately, atypical presentations of appendicitis appear to be the norm in elderly patients. Only 20% of elderly patients will have the classic findings of fever, anorexia, right lower quadrant pain, and leukocytosis [37]. Fever is seen in less than one-third of elderly patients at the time of presentation, right lower quadrant tenderness may be absent in 30%, and one-quarter will have a normal WBC count [38]. This may account for the staggering statistic that nearly one-quarter of elderly patients subsequently proven to have appendicitis are discharged home at the first ED visit [39].

It is no surprise then that the MANTRELS score underperforms in elderly patients. A study in 2001 showed that in 143 cases of surgically proven appendicitis, 12 cases would have been missed using the MANTRELS scoring system (i.e., MANTRELS score <5). Ten of the 12 cases were patients between the age of 60 and 80 years [40].

A higher than normal index of suspicion is required to accurately diagnose appendicitis in a timely fashion in elderly

Table 3.2 MANTRELS (Alvarado) Score for suspected acute appendicitis.

		Points
Symptoms	**M**igration	1
	Anorexia	1
	Nausea/vomiting	1
Signs	**T**enderness in right lower quadrant	2
	Rebound	1
	Elevated temperature (>100.4°F, >38.0°C)	1
Laboratory values	**L**eukocytosis (WBC >10,400 cells/ml)	2
	Shift to the left (>75% neutrophils on differential)	2
Total		10

Score: 5–6: possible appendicitis; 7–8: probable appendicitis; 9–10: very probable appendicitis.

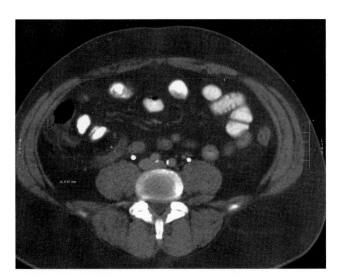

Figure 3.2 Acute appendicitis.
Axial view of CT scan demonstrating enlarged appendix that does not fill with contrast material, consistent with acute appendicitis.

patients. Low clinical suspicion or low MANTRELS score are not sufficient to exclude the diagnosis in this population. Liberal use of imaging with CT scan is encouraged early on in the course of elderly patients with abdominal pain (see Figure 3.2).

Conversely, another group of patients that the MANTRELS scoring system is less suited for is women. In this case, a high score has a lower positive predictive value than in children or men. Several studies have shown that even with scores of 7 or more, the percent of negative appendectomies is around one-third [41, 42]. In women, especially of child-bearing age, a high MANTRELS score may still require either confirmatory testing (i.e., CT scan) or testing to exclude other pelvic pathology (e.g., ultrasound or diagnostic laparoscopy) rather than proceeding directly to surgery.

Pitfall | Failure to appreciate atypical signs and symptoms in the elderly

The patient that presents in extremis with a rigid board-like abdomen presents little diagnostic dilemma for the EP. Stabilization, a call to the covering surgeon, and rapid mobilization of operative resources are quickly accomplished. There exist many patients however, that similarly require urgent or emergent surgical intervention, but present much less dramatically. This proportion increases considerably with advancing age. EPs may be falsely lulled into complacency when evaluating an elderly person with abdominal pain, as their presentation is often less dramatic. They often have atypical symptoms of disease, delays in presenting for evaluation, and a paucity of physical findings. Despite this, nearly one-third will require urgent surgical intervention, and fully one-half will require hospital admission [43]. Of those that

are discharged home, the recidivism rate is approximately one-third, significantly higher than younger patients with the same complaint. As noted above, appendicitis in the elderly is challenging to diagnose. Other difficult disease entities include PUD, biliary tract disease, and pancreatitis.

Peptic Ulcer Disease

> KEY FACT | One-half of all ulcers in the geriatric population will have a complication as their presenting symptom.

PUD remains a highly prevalent disease throughout the world. The mortality rate and number of hospitalizations is slowly decreasing, except in the geriatric population. Painless ulcers were found in 35% of patients older than 60 years with endoscopically proven PUD, compared with only 8% in those below the age of 60 years [44]. One-half of all ulcers in the geriatric population will have a complication as their presenting symptom [45]. Complications include hemorrhage, obstruction, or perforation/penetration.

Hemorrhagic complications of PUD are more common in the elderly. Twenty percent of cases have no prior symptoms of PUD. Elderly patients with hemorrhagic PUD are more likely to require blood transfusions, require surgery to control hemorrhage, and to rebleed [46]. To further complicate matters, the tachycardic response to hemorrhage may be absent due to intrinsic conduction system defects or masked by concomitant beta-blocker use.

Penetrations may be mistaken for pancreatitis or musculoskeletal back pain. In elderly patients, even anterior perforations may be difficult to diagnose. Acute onset of pain is found in only half the cases. Abdominal tenderness is often less severe, with overt rigidity seen in only 20% [47]. The yield of plain radiographs is much lower. Free intraperitoneal air is seen on only 40% of radiographs [48] (see Figure 3.3). This contributes to the increased mortality in elderly patients, which approaches 30%, compared to 10% in the general population [46]. Much of this mortality is directly attributable to delayed diagnosis. If the diagnosis is delayed by 24 h, the mortality rate increases 8-fold [48]. Some patients can be managed non-operatively, but all patients will require surgical consultation. A randomized, controlled trial of medical versus surgical treatment of perforated peptic ulcers showed that the group of patients older than 70 years was less likely to respond to conservative treatment [49].

Biliary Tract Disease

Cholelithiasis is an extremely common disease, affecting up to 10% of adults. Acute cholecystitis remains the most common reason for acute abdominal surgery in the elderly population [50]. The severity of biliary tract disease is much higher in the elderly. Complications including ascending

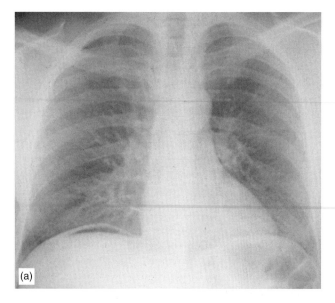

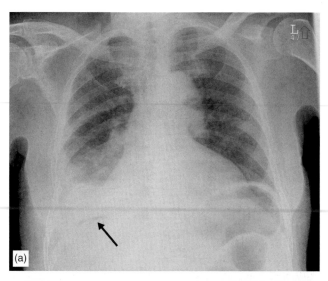

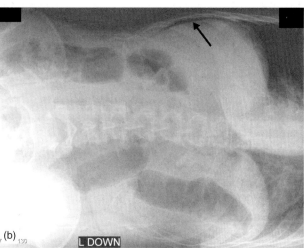

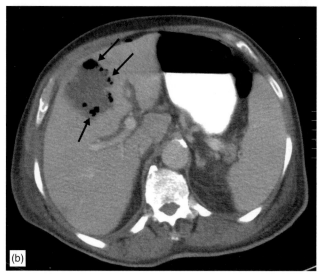

Figure 3.3 Free intraperitoneal air.
(a) This upright chest radiograph demonstrates free air under the right hemidiaphragm. This finding is highly specific for perforated viscus and almost always warrants emergent surgical intervention. (b) The left lateral decubitus radiograph is considered by many to have greater sensitivity for detection of free intraperitoneal air than even the upright chest radiograph. A small amount of air is noted between the edge of the liver and the costal margin (arrow). This type of radiograph is especially useful for patients whose medical condition prohibits them from sitting or standing upright for a chest radiograph.

Figure 3.4 Emphysematous cholecystitis.
(a) This upright plain radiograph demonstrates subtle evidence of air in the region of the hepatobiliary system (arrow), a finding that should always prompt consideration of two deadly conditions – acute mesenteric ischemia and emphysematous cholecystitis. The finding was overlooked, and after a delay, the final diagnosis of emphysematous cholecystitis was made by CT. (b) This is the CT of the same patient. The diagnosis of emphysematous cholecystitis was made based on the presence of air within the wall of the gallbladder (arrows).

cholangitis, gallbladder empyema, perforation, necrosis, and emphysematous cholecystitis are all more prevalent in this population [51]. The mortality rate from biliary tract disease in the elderly approaches 20%.

> KEY FACT | **One-half of elderly patients with AC will be afebrile … leukocytosis is absent in one-third and liver function tests are all normal in a significant percentage.**

AC in the elderly may lack the nausea and vomiting often seen in the younger patient. One-half of elderly patients with AC will be afebrile. This trend holds true even in the face of complications such as empyema, gangrene, or even frank perforation [52]. Leukocytosis is absent in one-third and liver function tests are all normal in a significant percentage. Although ultrasound and the sonographic Murphy's sign retain their sensitivity in the elderly, acalculous cholecystitis may be missed. This entity shows an increased prevalence in the elderly population.

Ascending cholangitis is seen more commonly in elderly patients, presumably due to the increased incidence of choledocholithiasis. Elderly patients often present in septic shock, with no prodrome of biliary colic-type symptoms. While conservative therapy with broad-spectrum antibiotics induces a response in 70–80% of cases, severely ill patients require emergent decompression. This may be open, percutaneous, or via endoscopic retrograde cholangiopancreatography (ERCP).

Gallbladder empyema is a complication of AC where the gallbladder fills with pus due to complete obstruction. It also is more common in the elderly, and carries a mortality rate of 25% [53]. In addition to antibiotics, urgent surgical decompression is required.

Emphysematous cholecystitis is an infection of the gallbladder wall by gas-forming organisms. The incidence rises with age, and it is associated with diabetes and peripheral vascular disease. It is the only biliary tract disease that is more common in men. Patients are typically toxic appearing. Diagnosis is made by visualizing air in the wall of the gallbladder on plain radiographs or CT (see Figure 3.4), or by the demonstration of "effervescent bile" on ultrasound. Surgery is the mainstay of therapy.

Pancreatitis

KEY FACT | **One-third of all cases of pancreatitis occur in the elderly … with mortality rates approaching 40%.**

AP is an inflammatory process where the pancreatic enzymes autodigest the gland. It ranges from a disease of mild severity to a life-threatening entity with hemorrhage or frank necrosis of the organ. It remains the most common non-surgical abdominal condition in the elderly population. The incidence of AP increases 200-fold among those aged 65 years and older [54]. One-third of all cases of pancreatitis occur in the elderly, and they tend to have a more severe course with mortality rates approaching 40% [55].

The clinical presentation in the elderly is quite varied. It may demonstrate the classic "boring" epigastric pain radiating to the back, or it may exhibit a hypermetabolic state resembling systemic inflammatory response syndrome. Unfortunately, in 10% of case of AP in the elderly, it merely presents with altered mental status and shock [45]. The risk of necrotizing pancreatitis is higher, especially as the patient's age approaches 80 years [56]. These patients are at high risk for rapid deterioration. As such, a low threshold for CT scanning in the elderly should be maintained, particularly if there are signs of impending sepsis. If CT scanning shows necrotizing pancreatitis and bacterial infection is established (usually through percutaneous aspiration), surgical intervention has been shown to be beneficial [57].

Pearls for Improving Patient Outcomes

- Always consider myocardial infarction as a cause of abdominal pain, especially in patients with traditional cardiac risk factors.
- Maintain a high index of suspicion for mesenteric ischemia in elderly patients and pursue early diagnostic imaging based on clinical suspicion alone.
- Do not assume that visualization of an IUP on ultrasound definitively rules out ectopic pregnancy in women undergoing ART. These patients are at high risk for heterotopic pregnancy.
- The MANTRELS scoring system is useful in selected patient populations, especially at both ends of the scoring spectrum. It should be used with caution (if at all) in elderly patients and women. Low MANTRELS scores in elderly patients should not preclude imaging with CT scan. High MANTRELS scores in women (especially of child-bearing age) should not reflexively trigger surgery, as they may still have other pelvic pathology not requiring operative treatment.
- Elderly patients often present with atypical signs and symptoms of common disease entities. A broad diagnostic net should be cast in these cases, and a period of observation with early follow-up should be routine, even if the patient appears well.

References

1. McCaig LF, Burt CW. National Hospital Ambulatory Medical Care Survey: 2003 emergency department summary. Advance data from vital and health statistics; no 358. Hyattsville, Maryland: National Center for Health Statistics. 2005.
2. Powers RD, Guertler AT. Abdominal pain in the ED: stability and change over 20 years. *Am J Emerg Med* 1995; 13:301–3.
3. Canto JG, Shlipak MG, Rogers WJ, Malmgren J, Frederick P, Lambrew CT, Ornato JP, Kiefe CI. Prevalence, clinical characteristics and mortality among patients with myocardial infarction presenting without chest pain. *J Am Med Assoc* 2000; 283:3223–9.
4. Lusiani L, Perrone A, Pesavento R, Conte G. Prevalence, clinical features and acute course of atypical myocardial infarction. *Angiology* 1994; 45:49–55.
5. Canto JG, Fincher C, Kiefe CI, Allison JJ, Li Q, Funkhouser E, et al. Atypical presentations among Medicare beneficiaries with unstable angina pectoris. *Am J Cardiol* 2002; 90:248–53.
6. Yu AC, Riegert-Johnson DL. A case of acute pancreatitis presenting with electrocardiographic signs of acute myocardial infarction. *Pancreatology* 2003; 3(6):515–17.
7. Albrecht C, Laws FA. ST segment elevation pattern of acute myocardial infarction induced by acute pancreatitis. *Cardiol Rev* 2003; 11(3):147–51.
8. Hung SC, Chiang CE, Chen JD, Ding PY. Images in cardiovascular medicine: pseudo-myocardial infarction. *Circulation* 2000; 101(25):2989–90.
9. Khairy P, Marsolais P. Pancreatitis with electrocardiographic changes mimicking acute myocardial infarction. *Can J Gastroenterol* 2001; 15(8):522–6.
10. Cafri C, Basok A, Katz A, Abuful A, Gilutz H, Battler A. Thrombolytic therapy in acute pancreatitis presenting as acute myocardial infarction. *Int J Cardiol* 1995; 49:279–81.

11. Wagner AM, Santolo M. A correct decision? *Lancet* 2002; 359(9301):157.

12. Stoney RJ, Cunningham CG. Acute mesenteric ischemia. *Surgery* 1993; 114:489–90.

13. Ruotolo RA, Evans SRT. Mesenteric ischemia in the elderly. *Clin Geriatr Med* 1999; 15:527–57.

14. Rhee RY, Gloviczki P, Mendonca CT, Petterson TM, Serry RD, Sarr MG, et al. Mesenteric venous thrombosis: still a lethal disease in the 1990s. *J Vasc Surg* 1994; 20:688–97.

15. Diamond S, Emmett M, Henrich WL. Bowel infarction as a cause of death in dialysis patients. *J Am Med Assoc* 1986; 256:2545.

16. Newman TS, Magnuson TH, Ahrendt SA, Smith-Meek MA, Bender JS. The changing face of mesenteric infarction. *Am Surg* 1998; 64:611.

17. Sai-Sudhakar CB, Al-Hakeem M, MacArthur JD, Sumpio BE. Mesenteric ischemia secondary to cocaine abuse: case reports and literature review. *Am J Gastroenterol* 1997; 92:1053.

18. Boley SJ, Sprayregen S, Siegelman SJ, Veith FJ. Initial results from an aggressive roentgenologic and surgical approach to acute mesenteric ischemia. *Surgery* 1977; 82:848.

19. Clark RA, Gallant TE. Acute mesenteric ischemia: angiographic spectrum. *Am J Roentgenol* 1984; 142:555.

20. Lobo Martinez E, Carvajosa E, Sacco O, Martinez Molina E. Embolectomy in mesenteric ischemia. *Rev Esp Enferm Dig* 1993; 83:351.

21. Bradbury MS, Kavanaugh PV, Chen MY, Weber TM, Bechtold RE. Noninvasive assessment of portomesenteric venous thrombosis: current concepts and imaging strategies. *J Comput Assist Tomogr* 2002; 26:392–404.

22. Hellinger JC. Evaluating mesenteric ischemia with multidetector-row CT angiography. *Tech Vasc Interv Radiol* 2004; 7(3):160–6.

23. Simon BC, Snoey ER. Ultrasound in emergency and ambulatory medicine. St. Louis: Mosby; 1997.

24. Reece EA, Petrie RH, Sirmans MF, Finster M, Todd WD. Combined intrauterine and extrauterine gestations: a review. *Am J Obstet Gynecol* 1983; 146:323–30.

25. Habana A, Dokras A, Giraldo J, et al. Cornual heterotopic pregnancy: contemporary management options. *Am J Obstet Gynecol* 2000; 182:1264–70.

26. Sotrel G, Rao R, Scommegna A. Heterotopic pregnancy following clomid treatment. *J Reprod Med* 1976; 16:78–80.

27. Botta G, Fortunato N, Merlino G. Heterotopic pregnancy following administration of human menopausal gonadotropin in vitro fertilization and embryo transfer: two case reports and review of the literature. *Eur J Obstet Gynecol Reprod Biol* 1995; 59:2112–15.

28. Sucov A, Deveau L, Feola P, et al. Heterotopic pregnancy after in vitro fertilization. *Am J Emerg Med* 1995; 13:641–3.

29. Jerrard D, Tso E, Salik R, Barish RA. Unsuspected heterotopic pregnancy in a woman without risk factors. *Am J Emerg Med* 1992; 10:58–60.

30. Dart R, McLean S, Dart L. Isolated fluid in the cul-de-sac: how well does it predict ectopic pregnancy? *Am J Emerg Med* 2002; 20:1–4.

31. Breyer MJ, Costantino TG. Heterotopic gestation: Another possibility for the emergency bedside ultrasonographer to consider. *J Emerg Med* 2004; 26(1):81–4.

32. Somers MP, Spears M, Maynard AS, Syverud SA. Ruptured heterotopic pregnancy presenting with relative bradycardia in a woman not receiving reproductive assistance. *Ann Emerg Med* 2004; 43:382–5.

33. Irvin TT. Abdominal pain: a surgical audit of 1190 emergency admissions. *Br J Surg* 1989; 76:1121–5.

34. Schwartz SI. Appendix. In: Schwartz SI (ed.), *Principles of surgery*, 6th edn. New York: McGraw Hill, 1994, pp. 1307–18.

35. Yamini D, Hernan V, Bongard F, et al. Perforated appendicitis: is it truly a surgical emergency? *Am Surg* 1995; 221:279–82.

36. Alvarado A. A practical score for the early diagnosis of acute appendicitis. *Ann Emerg Med* 1986; 15:557–64.

37. Horattas MC, Guyton DP, Wu D. A reappraisal of appendicitis in the elderly. *Am J Surg* 1990; 160:291–3.

38. Storm-Dickerson TL, Horattas MC. What have we learned over the past 20 years about appendicitis in the elderly? *Am J Surg* 2003; 185:198–201.

39. Rogers J. Abdominal Pain: Forsight. Dallas: American College of Emergency Physicians; Issue 3, Dec 1986.

40. Gwynn LK. The diagnosis of acute appendicitis: Clinical assessment versus computed tomography evaluation. *J Emerg Med* 2001; 21(2):119–23.

41. Malik AA, Wani NA. Continuing diagnostic challenge of acute appendicitis: evaluation through modified Alvarado score. *Aust NZ J Surg* 1998; 68:504–5.

42. Kalan M, Talbot D, Cunliffe WJ, Rich AJ. Evaluation of the modified Alvarado score in the diagnosis of acute appendicitis: a prospective study. *Ann Roy Coll Surg Engl* 1994; 76:418–419.

43. Brewer RJ, Golden GT, Hitsch DC, et al. Abdominal pain: an analysis of 1,000 consecutive cases in a university hospital emergency room. *Am J Surg* 1976; 131:219–24.

44. Leverat M. Peptic ulcer disease in patients over 60: experience in 287 cases. *Am J Dig Dis* 1966; 11:279–85.

45. Caesar R. Dangerous complaints: The acute geriatric abdomen. *Emerg Med Report* 1994; 15:191–202.

46. Borum ML. Peptic-ulcer disease in the elderly. *Clin Geriatr Med* 1999; 15(3):457–71.

47. Fenyo G. Acute abdominal disease in the elderly: experience from two series in Stockholm. *Am J Surg* 1982; 143:751–4.

48. Wakayama T. Risk factors influencing the short-term results of gastroduodenal perforation. *Surg Today* 1994; 24(8):681–7.

49. Crofts TJ, Park KG, Steele RJ. A randomized trial of nonoperative treatment for perforated peptic ulcer. *New Engl J Med* 1989; 320(15):970–3.

50. Rosenthal RA, Anderson DK: Surgery in the elderly: observations on the pathophysiology and treatment of cholelithiasis. *Exp Gerontol* 1993; 28:459–72.

51. Bedirli A. Factors effecting the complications in the natural history of acute cholecystitis. *Hepatogastroenterol* 2001; 48(41): 1275–8.

52. Morrow DJ, Thompson J, Wilson SE. Acute cholecystitis in the elderly. *Arch Surg* 1978; 113:1149–52.

53. Sen M, Williamson RCN. Acute cholecystitis: surgical management. *Balliere's Clin Gastroenterol* 1991; 5:817–37.

54. Martin SP, Ulrich CD. Pancreatic disease in the elderly. *Clin Geriatr Med* 1999; 15(3):579–605.

55. Hoffman E, Perez E. Acute pancreatitis in the upper age groups. *Gastroenterol* 1959; 36:675–85.

56. Paajanen H. AP in patients over 80 years. *Eur J Surg* 1996; 162(6):471–5.

57. Bradley EL III, Allen K. A prospective longitudinal study of observation versus surgical intervention in the management of necrotizing pancreatitis. *Am J Surg* 1991; 161:19–24.

Chapter 4 | Management of Patients with Acute Back Pain in the ED

Michael E. Winters

Introduction

Up to 90% of adults will have at least one episode of back pain during their lifetime [1]. In the US alone, approximately 15 million patients present each year to a physician with acute back pain [2]. Many of these patients arrive at local emergency departments (ED) seeking evaluation and symptom relief. In fact, back pain accounts for almost 2% of all ED visits per year [3]. Thankfully, 90–95% of patients presenting with acute back pain have non-life-threatening etiologies [4]. Although most patients cannot be given an exact diagnosis, nearly all recover within 4–6 weeks [1, 5].

In the remaining 5–10% of patients, acute back pain is a manifestation of serious pathology. Thoracic aortic dissection, abdominal aortic aneurysm, spinal epidural abscess, spinal epidural metastasis, and spinal cord compressive syndromes may all initially present with a complaint of acute back pain. These "back pain emergencies" are missed in a significant percentage of patients upon initial evaluation. As a result of delays in diagnosis and treatment, patients with these conditions continue to have unacceptably high morbidity and mortality. Although challenging, it is crucial that emergency physicians identify patients with acute back pain with a potentially life-threatening disorder.

This chapter will focus on common pitfalls in the ED evaluation of patients with acute back pain. With this information, the emergency physician can more effectively detect and treat patients with potentially catastrophic causes of back pain.

Pitfall | Over-reliance on the "Classic" Clinical Presentations of Aortic Dissection, Rupturing Abdominal Aortic Aneurysm, Spinal Epidural Abscess, and Pulmonary Embolism

In emergency medicine, it is well recognized that the textbook clinical presentations of disease are often the exception rather than the rule. This holds true for the clinical presentations of several dangerous back pain emergencies [6]. The emergency physician must be able to diagnose these life-threatening disorders even in the absence of "classic" presentations.

> **KEY FACT** | The "classic" description of aortic dissection pain is absent in 2/3 of cases.

The classic clinical description of aortic dissection is the sudden onset of ripping chest pain that radiates to the interscapular region. In reality, this textbook description is present in less than one-third of patients with aortic dissection [6]. Although the abrupt onset of pain is reported in 85% of patients, many will not describe their pain as either ripping or tearing [7, 8]. Patients with aortic dissection often describe their pain as either sharp, pressure-like, pleuritic, or even burning [7]. In addition to a variety of descriptions of pain, patients with aortic dissection often report varying locations of pain. Isolated back pain, especially thoracic, is common in dissections of the descending aorta.

Textbook physical examination findings of aortic dissection include hypertension, pulse deficits, blood pressure differentials, and a new diastolic murmur. These classic abnormalities are inconsistent and unreliable findings in patients with dissection. Up to one-third of patients with an acute aortic dissection are normotensive upon evaluation [9]. Although considered specific for aortic dissection, a pulse deficit occurs in just 25–38% of cases [6, 9] and its absence cannot be used to exclude the diagnosis of aortic dissection. Bilateral blood pressure measurements are frequently obtained in cases of suspected aortic dissection. A difference of 20 mmHg or more is considered significant. However, 20% of normal individuals have blood pressure differentials greater than 20 mmHg, thereby lowering the specificity of this finding [10–12]. The sensitivity of a new diastolic murmur in the detection of aortic dissection is reportedly just 28% [6]. Thus, it is easy to see how the clinical examination is inadequate for diagnosing or excluding an acute aortic dissection [9]. For the emergency physician, suspicion for aortic dissection begins by identifying risk factors for aortic pathology. A thorough risk factor analysis for aortic disease must be performed in any patient presenting with acute back pain. Risk factor assessment has been shown to increase the rate of diagnosis of aortic catastrophes [10]. Thoracic aortic dissection must be considered in any patient with risk factors for the same (discussed below) who presents with the abrupt onset of severe thoracic back pain.

> KEY FACT | **Rupturing abdominal aortic aneurysm often presents with symptoms mimicking renal colic, diverticulitis, and musculoskeletal pain.**

The textbook triad of rupturing abdominal aortic aneurysm consists of abdominal pain, hypotension, and a pulsatile abdominal mass. Unfortunately, less than 20% of patients with a rupturing aneurysm present with this triad [13]. It is important for the emergency physician to recognize that a rupturing abdominal aortic aneurysm can present with left lower quadrant pain, flank pain, or isolated back pain. As a result, many patients with a ruptured aneurysm are misdiagnosed as having diverticulitis, nephrolithiasis, pyelonephritis, or musculoskeletal strain [13]. Misdiagnosis leads to significant morbidity and mortality. Mortality rates as high as 75% have been reported when patients with a rupturing abdominal aortic aneurysm are initially misdiagnosed [10]. In addition to recognizing back or flank pain as the initial presenting symptom, the emergency physician must also understand the limitations of physical examination.

> KEY FACT | **Abdominal palpation is insensitive for detecting abdominal aortic aneurysm.**

The sensitivity of abdominal palpation for an aneurysm ranges from 45% to 97% [13]. Sensitivity increases with increasing sizes of aneurysm, however, nearly 25% of abdominal aneurysms greater than 5 cm cannot be palpated [13]. Similar to aortic dissection, suspicion for an abdominal aortic aneurysm begins with a thorough risk factor assessment. A rupturing aneurysm must be considered in any elderly patient with acute back, or flank pain, who has risk factors for an abdominal aortic aneurysm.

> KEY FACT | **Because the vast majority of patients with spinal epidural abscesses present atypically, assessment of patients for risk factors for this disease is essential for identifying it prior to the onset of irreversible neurological sequelae.**

Spinal epidural abscess is classically associated with the triad of fever, back pain, and neurologic deficits. Although these symptoms are helpful if present, this triad occurs in as few as 13% of patients [14]. Up to 75% of patients with a spinal epidural abscess will be afebrile and up to two-thirds of patients will have a normal initial neurologic exam [14]. As a result, patients with spinal epidural abscess incur significant diagnostic delays. Often, patients with spinal epidural abscess have multiple ED visits before the diagnosis is made. Since rapid neurologic deterioration can occur, it is imperative that

the emergency physician identify patients with a spinal epidural abscess. Rather than relying on the presence of fever and back pain, the emergency physician should focus on identifying risk factors for spinal epidural abscess in any patient with acute back pain. It is reported that risk factor assessment offers the highest sensitivity and negative predictive value in identifying patients with spinal epidural abscess before the onset of neurologic symptoms [14].

The clinical presentation of pulmonary embolism is classically described as the acute onset of pleuritic chest pain associated with dyspnea and hemoptysis. Atypical presentations of pulmonary embolism, however, are common. Thoracic back pain is a recognized presentation of pulmonary embolism [15]. In addition to aortic catastrophes and infectious etiologies, the emergency physician should include a risk factor assessment for venous thromboembolic disease when confronted with the patient with acute thoracic back pain.

Pitfall | **Failure to Perform a Risk Factor Assessment for Serious Etiologies of Back Pain**

Since the majority of patients with back pain have benign etiologies, identification of the patient in whom to pursue an extensive diagnostic workup is challenging. Suspicion for serious pathology begins with an assessment of patient risk factors for disease. Unfortunately, many physicians fail to perform a risk factor profile in patients presenting with back pain. In fact, failure to inquire about risk factors is one of the most common reasons cited in cases of missed aortic dissection [10]. Thus, it is imperative that the emergency physician inquire about risk factors, perform a risk factor assessment, and guide the workup accordingly. In many cases, risk factors may be the only clue to serious underlying pathology.

> KEY FACT | **Pregnancy is an often overlooked risk factor for aortic dissection.**

Risk factors for aortic catastrophes are well established and include male gender, older age, hypertension, connective tissue disorders, chromosomal syndromes, smoking, and inflammatory conditions of the aorta [16]. Additional risk factors for aortic dissection include a bicuspid aortic valve, coarctation, aortic instrumentation, decelerating trauma, and pregnancy [16]. In fact, over 50% of aortic dissections in women less than 40 years of age occur during pregnancy, most often during the third trimester and the initial stages of labor [16]. Aortic dissection must be considered in the differential diagnosis of any pregnant patient presenting during the third trimester or labor with the abrupt onset of severe back pain.

> KEY FACT | **Aortic dissection must be excluded in hypertensive patients with back pain and a history of recent cocaine use.**

Lastly, the emergency physician must always inquire about the use of illicit substances in patients with back pain. Cocaine use is an established risk factor for aortic dissection, particularly of the descending aorta, in otherwise healthy individuals [16]. Hypertensive patients presenting with the abrupt onset of back pain in the setting of cocaine use should be imaged to exclude acute aortic dissection.

> KEY FACT | **Patients with back pain using injection drugs must have diagnostic imaging to definitively exclude spinal epidural abscess.**

Although traditionally taught as a disease of older individuals, spinal epidural abscess can affect patients of any age. Risk factors for spinal epidural abscess include diabetes mellitus, alcoholism, chronic renal failure, corticosteroid therapy, human immunodeficiency virus/acquired immunodeficiency syndrome, and intravenous drug use [17]. Intravenous drug use is considered one of the primary risk factors for spinal epidural abscess, accounting for over 50% of cases in some populations [18]. Any patient with back pain who uses intravenous drugs must be considered to have a spinal epidural abscess until proven otherwise. Regardless of the location of pain, these patients require imaging to exclude an epidural abscess. It is also important for the emergency physician to inquire about recent invasive procedures. Back pain that develops in the setting of a recent procedure, especially one known to have a high incidence of bacteremia, is highly suspicious for either vertebral osteomyelitis or spinal epidural abscess [1].

> KEY FACT | **Spinal metastases must be considered in patients with back pain and a history of malignancy, regardless of the type.**

Epidural spinal cord compression is a true medical emergency that cannot be missed. Over 90% of cases are due to spinal epidural metastases. The primary risk factor for spinal epidural metastases is a history of malignancy. Although prostate, breast, and lung cancer most commonly cause bony metastases, it is important to realize that any systemic malignancy can metastasize to the spine. Lymphoma, renal cell cancer, gastrointestinal malignancies, and multiple myeloma are frequently overlooked, yet account for a significant percentage of cases. Spinal epidural metastases with resultant spinal cord compression must be considered in any patient with back pain and a history of malignancy. Additional etiologies for spinal cord compression include massive midline disc herniation, spinal hematoma, epidural abscess, traumatic compression, and transverse myelitis [19].

Pitfall | **Failure to Perform a Complete Neurologic Exam**

Arguably, the most important portion of the physical examination in patients with back pain is the neurologic examination. In many cases, subtle neurologic deficits are the only indication of serious pathology, namely spinal cord compression. Unfortunately, many physicians either fail to perform a complete neurologic exam or fail to appropriately document their findings. In a review of missed cases of spinal epidural abscess, Davis et al. report that, in each case, minimal notation was made with regards to the neurologic exam [14]. Exams were documented as either "nonfocal" or "normal" without reference to the motor, sensory, deep tendon reflex, rectal, or cerebellar components.

> KEY FACT | **It is imperative to perform a complete neurologic examination including, when indicated, a rectal examination and post-void residual measurement.**

The importance of performing a complete neurologic exam cannot be overstated. Any patient with acute back pain and neurologic deficits requires emergent diagnostic imaging. In cases of spinal cord compression, motor deficits are the most common neurologic finding and are present in up to 85% of patients [20]. The emergency physician must pay close attention to the motor examination of the lower extremities. Appropriate examination should include an assessment of hip flexion and extension, leg flexion and extension, ankle dorsiflexion and inversion, and great toe dorsiflexion. In cases of thoracic spinal cord compression, the iliopsoas muscles are preferentially affected, producing weakness of the proximal lower extremities when testing hip flexion [20]. Sensory abnormalities occur slightly less often than motor deficits, whereas bowel and/or bladder dysfunction is a late finding in patients with epidural spinal cord compression [20]. Any patient with a report of fecal retention or incontinence and/or saddle anesthesia must have a rectal examination performed *and documented*. Additional indications for rectal examination include severe pain and/or the presence of any neurologic deficit. In addition to the rectal examination, patients with suspected spinal cord compression should have a post-void residual measurement. A post-void residual greater than 100–200 ml is indicative of acute urinary retention. Regardless of a history of prostatic abnormalities, any patient with acute back pain and an abnormal post-void residual should be suspected of having spinal cord compression until proven otherwise. Acute urinary retention is reported to have 90% sensitivity and 95% specificity for cauda equina syndrome [19].

Pitfall | Failure to Recognize the Limitations of Plain Radiography in Excluding a Back Pain Emergency

> KEY FACT | There is virtually no indication for plain radiography in the evaluation of nontraumatic back pain.

Given their low cost and ready availability, plain radiographs are frequently obtained in the evaluation of patients with acute back pain. In the setting of trauma, plain films can be useful to exclude fracture or dislocation. However, plain films are often erroneously utilized to exclude other potential back pain emergencies, such as spinal metastases or vertebral osteomyelitis. For vertebral metastases, plain radiographs are the least sensitive of all imaging modalities [4]. The pooled sensitivity of plain radiographs for spinal metastases is just 60% [4]. Furthermore, up to 17% of patients with epidural spinal cord compression due to metastatic disease have normal plain radiographs [20]. For the patient presenting with acute back pain and neurologic deficits, plain films should not be relied upon as the sole imaging modality to exclude spinal epidural metastases or spinal cord compression.

Plain radiographs are equally insensitive in the diagnosis of infectious etiologies of back pain, namely osteomyelitis and spinal epidural abscess. Abnormalities that indicate a potential infectious etiology include endplate erosion, loss of vertebral disc height, and bony lysis, but these abnormalities usually take several weeks to develop [4]. Thus, patients with infectious etiologies of back pain may have entirely normal plain films. For osteomyelitis, <33% of patients will have an abnormality on plain film during the first 7–10 days [21]. The overall sensitivity and specificity of plain radiographs for osteomyelitis or epidural abscess is 82% and 57%, respectively, and therefore cannot be used solely to rule out spinal infection [4]. Given the potential for rapid neurologic deterioration, once these disease entities are suspected, definitive diagnostic imaging is indicated rather than false reassurance with plain radiography.

Pitfall | Failure to Consider Aortic Catastrophes in Patients with Acute Back Pain and Neurologic Symptoms

The emergency physician must be knowledgeable regarding atypical presentations of aortic dissection and abdominal aortic aneurysm. It is imperative to recognize that aortic catastrophes can present with back pain and focal neurologic abnormalities. In fact, neurologic deficits are found in 18–36% of patients with aortic dissection [10]. Deficits seen in patients with aortic dissection range from acute stroke to unilateral lower extremity numbness. Unilateral lower extremity deficits are caused by involvement of the great radicular artery, a branch of the descending aorta. Thoracic aortic dissection must be excluded in any patient with sudden thoracic back pain and focal neurologic deficits.

> KEY FACT | Hematoma surrounding an abdominal aortic aneurysm can cause weakness of hip and knee flexion.

For rupturing abdominal aortic aneurysm, up to 5% of patients will have associated neurologic deficits [10]. It is believed that an expanding retroperitoneal hematoma causes direct nerve compression. Since the femoral and obturator nerves are the most susceptible to compression, patients present with weakness of hip and knee flexion [10]. The emergency physician must consider aortic catastrophes in the differential diagnosis of patients presenting with back pain and neurologic deficits.

Pitfall | Failure to Recognize the Limitations of Laboratory Studies in the Evaluation of Patients with Suspected Spinal Epidural Abscess or Vertebral Osteomyelitis

> KEY FACT | Lab studies cannot be used exclusively to rule out an infectious cause of back pain.

When considering an infectious etiology of back pain, physicians frequently rely on the presence of a leukocytosis to guide further evaluation. This finding is variable in infectious causes of back pain. White blood cell counts above 12,000/mm^3 are seen in just 40% of patients with spinal infection [22]. In addition, the presence of a left shift has been shown to be unreliable in the detection of an infectious etiology [17]. Emergency physicians should never exclude the possibility of a spinal infection based upon a normal white blood cell count.

In contrast to the peripheral white blood cell count, inflammatory markers, such as the erythrocyte sedimentation rate and C-reactive protein, have been shown to be useful in the identification of patients with a spinal infection. These markers are elevated in approximately 90% of patients with an infectious cause of back pain [21]. Up to 10% of patients can have normal levels, therefore, these markers should not be used as the sole criterion for excluding spinal infection.

Pitfall | Inadequate Radiographic Imaging in the Diagnosis of Spinal Cord Compression and Spinal Epidural Abscess

> KEY FACT | Magnetic resonance imaging is currently the only imaging modality that can be used to exclude spinal cord compression or abscess.

Emergency physicians recognize that spinal cord compression is a true emergency. Therefore, once the diagnosis is suspected, emergent imaging must be obtained. As discussed, plain films may be falsely negative in up to 17% of patients with cord compression [20]. Bone scanning, computed tomography, and positron-emission tomography have all been used in the evaluation of patients with spinal cord compression. These modalities, however, have not been shown to be superior to magnetic resonance imaging. Magnetic resonance imaging is the imaging modality of choice when diagnosing or excluding spinal cord compression. The overall diagnostic accuracy of magnetic resonance imaging for spinal cord compression is 95% [20]. For patients suspected of cord compression due to metastatic disease, magnetic resonance imaging of the entire spine is recommended, as compression can occur at multiple levels [23].

Definitive diagnostic imaging must also be obtained when considering the diagnosis of spinal epidural abscess. Magnetic resonance imaging is the most sensitive modality for identifying and characterizing spinal epidural abscess. Magnetic resonance imaging accurately defines the extent of an abscess, highlights any surrounding inflammation, evaluates the degree of thecal sac compression, and aids in the planning of surgical drainage. Sensitivity and specificity of magnetic resonance imaging for spinal infection is 96% and 92%, respectively [4]. Computed tomography myelography remains an option for patients unable to undergo magnetic resonance imaging; however, this procedure is invasive and can result in transmission of the infection into the subarachnoid space. Currently, there is no data on the accuracy of computed tomography without myelography in the diagnosis of osteomyelitis or spinal epidural abscess [4]. Similar to spinal epidural metastases, infectious etiologies of back pain can occur at multiple spinal levels, especially in the patient abusing intravenous drugs. A magnetic resonance scan that images only isolated sections of the spine will undoubtedly miss lesions at other spinal levels. Therefore, the *entire spine* should be imaged when evaluating patients for spinal epidural abscess.

Pitfall | **Inadequate Antibiotic Treatment in Patients with Infectious Etiologies of Back Pain**

Although optimal management of spinal epidural abscess remains controversial, all patients with an infectious etiology of acute back pain require prompt antibiotic administration. Ideally, antibiotics are given after tissue cultures are obtained. Because patients can develop rapid, irreversible

> KEY FACT | **In suspected spinal infection, antibiotics such as a third-generation cephalosporin plus a penicillinase-resistant penicillin or vancomycin should be administered as soon as possible after cultures are obtained.**

neurologic deterioration, it is crucial for the emergency physician to begin antibiotic therapy promptly.

Staphylococcal aureus is the most common isolate in cases of osteomyelitis and epidural abscess, but up to one-third of cases are caused by gram-negative organisms [24, 25]. Therefore, initial antibiotic coverage must be broad spectrum and effective against both gram-positive and gram-negative organisms. Acceptable regimens include a penicillinase-resistant penicillin plus a third-generation cephalosporin, or in cases of suspected methicillin-resistant *Staphylococcal aureus*, vancomycin and a third-generation cephalosporin [21].

Pitfall | **Failure to Initiate Prompt Treatment in the Patient with Spinal Cord Compression**

> KEY FACT | **Parenteral pain medications and dexamethasone (10 mg followed by 6 mg every 4 h) should be administered to patients with suspected spinal cord compression.**

Definitive treatment of epidural spinal cord compression requires a multi-disciplinary approach. *Once the diagnosis is suspected*, appropriate consultation must be obtained. Often, this involves consultation with neurosurgery, orthopedic surgery, and radiation oncology. While awaiting definitive treatment, the emergency physician must provide supportive care. Analgesics and corticosteroids are an important component of that supportive care. Corticosteroids have been shown to reduce edema, inhibit further inflammatory damage, and delay the progression of neurologic deficits [20]. Recent randomized trials have demonstrated that, in the case of cord compression due to metastatic disease, patients who received corticosteroids were more likely to be ambulatory at long-term follow up [23, 26]. Dexamethasone is the corticosteroid of choice given its low cost and relatively low mineralocorticoid activity [23]. Currently, there is no concensus on the optimal dose. Dosing regimens in the literature have ranged from 16 to 100 mg/day [20]. An acceptable regimen consists of an initial dose of 10 mg of dexamethasone, followed by 6 mg every 4 h.

Pitfall | **Failure to Promptly Refer Patients with an Acute Motor Radiculopathy**

> KEY FACT | **Patients with radiculopathy and motor deficits should have urgent neurosurgical referral.**

Only 2–3% of patients presenting with acute low back pain will have evidence of a lumbar radiculopathy [1]. Although there are many potential etiologies, the most common cause of a radiculopathy is an acute disc herniation. The size, level, and location of herniation determine a patient's symptoms and physical examination findings. In contrast to the patient with low back pain and a normal physical exam, those with a lumbar motor radiculopathy may require early surgical treatment. The most important factor in determining whether an early surgical procedure is needed is the presence of significant weakness [27]. If the weakness is substantial, delaying surgery could result in a permanent deficit. Therefore, it is incumbent upon the emergency physician to ensure that the patient with an acute lumbar motor radiculopathy is seen within seven days of their ED visit. Urgent magnetic resonance imaging, as well as neurosurgical referral, is needed to ensure optimal outcomes.

Pearls for Improving Patient Outcomes

- "Classic" presentations are the exception rather than the rule in back pain emergencies and they often present with symptoms mimicking other disease.
- Risk factors assessment is crucial to help identify patients requiring emergent imaging.
- Pregnancy is a risk factor for aortic dissection.
- A history of drug use should heighten suspicion for emergent causes of back pain.
- Patients with back pain require a careful neurological examination to identify those requiring emergent treatment.
- Plain films of the back are almost never indicated for nontraumatic back pain.
- Magnetic resonance imaging is currently the only test that can exclude spinal cord compression or abscess.
- For spinal infections, early administration of appropriate antibiotics is crucial.
- Steroids are indicated for patients with spinal cord compression.
- Patients with radicular symptoms and motor deficits should have urgent neurosurgical referral.

References

1. Della-Giustina DA. Orthopedic emergencies: emergency department evaluation and treatment of back pain. *Emerg Med Clin N Am* 1999; 17(4):877–93.
2. Hart L, Deyo R, Churkin D. Physician office visits for low back pain. *Spine* 1995; 20:11–19.
3. 1995 National Hospital Ambulatory Care Survey. National Center for Health Statistics, Center for Disease Control and Prevention, Hyattsville, Maryland.
4. Jarvik JG, Deyo RD. Diagnostic evaluation of low back pain with emphasis on imaging. *Ann Intern Med* 2002; 137:586–97.
5. Bigos S, Bowyer O, Braen G, et al. Acute low back problems in adults. In: *Clinical Practice Guideline*, Quick Reference Number 14, Rockville MD, U.S. Department of Health and Human Services, Public Health Service, Agency for Health Care Policy and Research. AHCPR Pub No. 95-0643. 1994.
6. Haro LH, Krajicek M, Lobl JK. Challenges, controversies, and advances in aortic catastrophes. *Emerg Med Clin N Am* 2005; 23:1159–77.
7. Sullivan PR, Wolfson AB, Leckey RD, Burke JL. Diagnosis of acute thoracic aortic dissection in the emergency department. *Am J Emerg Med* 2000; 18:46–50.
8. Hagan PG, Nienaber CA, Isselbacher EM, et al. The International Registry of Acute Aortic Dissection (IRAD): new insights into an old disease. *J Am Med Assoc* 2000; 283;897–903.
9. Knaut AL, Cleveland JC. Aortic emergencies. *Emerg Med Clin N Am* 2003; 21:817–45.
10. Rogers RL, McCormack R. Aortic disasters. *Emerg Med Clin N Am* 2004; 22:887–908.
11. Lane D, Beevers M, Barnes N, et al. Inter-arm differences in blood pressure: when are they clinically relevant? *J Hypertension* 2002; 20:1089.
12. Pesola GR, Pesola HR, Lin M, et al. The normal difference in bilateral blood indirect blood pressure recordings in hypertensive individuals. *Acad Emerg Med* 2002; 9:342–5.
13. Carpenter CR. Abdominal palpation for the diagnosis of abdominal aortic aneurysm. *Ann Emerg Med* 2005; 4:556–8.
14. Davis DP, Wold RM, Patel RJ, et al. The clinical presentation and impact of diagnostic delays on emergency department patients with spinal epidural abscess. *J Emerg Med* 2004; 26:285–91.
15. Laack TA, Goyal DG. Pulmonary embolism: an unsuspected killer. *Emerg Med Clin N Am* 2004; 22:961–83.
16. Khan IA, Nair CK. Clinical, diagnostic, and management perspectives of aortic dissection. *Chest* 2002; 122:311–28.
17. Soehle M, Wallenfang T. Spinal epidural abscess: clinical manifestations, prognostic factors, and outcomes. *Neurosurgery* 2002; 51:79–87.
18. Calder KK, Severyn FA. Surgical emergencies in the intravenous drug user. *Emerg Med Clin N Am* 2003; 21:1089–116.
19. Small SA, Perron AD, Brady WJ. Orthopedic pitfalls: cauda equina syndrome. *Am J Emerg Med* 2005; 23:159–63.
20. Prasad D, Schiff D. Malignant spinal-cord compression. *Lancet Oncol* 2005; 6:15–24.
21. Perron AD, Brady WJ, Miller MD. Orthopedic pitfalls: osteomyelitis. *Am J Emerg Med* 2003; 21:61–7.
22. Lurie JD, Gerber PD, Sox HC. A pain in the back. *New Engl J Med* 2000; 343:723–6.
23. Schiff D. Spinal cord compression. *Neurol Clin N Am* 2003; 21:67–86.
24. Lu C, Chang W, Lui C, et al. Adult spinal epidural abscess: clinical features and prognostic factors. *Clin Neurol and Neurosurg* 2002; 104:306–10.
25. Tunkel AR, Pradham SK. Central nervous system infections in injection drug users. *Infect Dis Clin N Am* 2002; 16:589–605.
26. Sorensen PS, Helweg-Larsen S, Mouridsen H, et al. Effect of high-dose dexamethasone in carcinomatous metastatic spinal cord compression treated with radiotherapy: a randomized trial. *Eur J Cancer* 1994; 30A:22–7.
27. Devereaux MW. Low back pain. *Prim Care Clin Office Pract* 2004; 31:33–51.

Chapter 5 | Headache Management

Stephen Schenkel

Introduction

In the course of a single year, 90% of people will experience headache [1]. Headaches account for fully 1–2% of emergency department (ED) visits, and the causes are myriad [2]. The International Headache Society classification breaks headaches into 13 categories. Still of those patients with headache that find their way to the ED, perhaps as few as 1% will be found to have a serious underlying neurologic disorder [3]. In Emergency medicine (EM), identifying a specific cause of headache is less important than differentiating those headaches with associated morbidity and treating them appropriately. The potential for encountering pitfalls is large. Headache is a common ED complaint and only a minority of patients have serious underlying pathology. The pitfalls are many. It is easy to err in diagnosis and miss the opportunity to treat the one or two seriously ill patients from every hundred who present with headache.

Pitfall | Failure to identify "red flag" features of headaches

Because headaches present frequently to the ED and the majority are benign, the emergency physician (EP) can easily be lulled into complacency. Determining which headaches require neuroimaging can be a challenge. While not all serious headaches will present with "red flags," failure to elicit high-risk features will increase the likelihood of missing serious pathology.

The classic "do not miss" headaches are a simple, short list: meningitis, brain tumor or other mass lesion, and intracranial hemorrhage. The most effective and commonly available initial diagnostic tests to evaluate for these four items are computed tomography (CT) and spinal fluid analysis after lumbar puncture (LP), but it is inefficient and wasteful to simply perform a CT and LP on everyone who presents with headache. Downsides include time, discomfort, false positive results, radiation exposure, infection, and – in the ultimate irony of LP for headache – post-dural puncture headache. Determining who should receive diagnostic imaging and/or LP is crucial to the management of this complaint.

> KEY FACT | Headaches in the elderly, patients with a history of malignancy or immunosuppression, those that represent a change from a patient's typical headache pattern, or those that are associated with abnormal neurologic findings should prompt consideration for further diagnostic testing.

It is important to determine whether the presenting headache represents a change from the typical headache pattern experienced by the patient. Likewise, headaches in patients with cancer, immunosuppression, the elderly, or with associated neurologic findings should raise concern and prompt further investigations.

It may be difficult to make the distinction between the need for emergency scanning versus that which can wait a few days or even weeks for follow-up. For many, practicing in an environment where a head CT is readily available, and where follow-up may be more difficult, the distinction becomes less important. Though dependent on social considerations (such as the likelihood of follow-up and resource availability), headaches with associated "red flags" should have as complete a workup in the ED as possible (Table 5.1).

Table 5.1 "Red flag" indications for ED neuroimaging (CT or MRI) [3, 11].

- First or worst headache of life, especially if rapid onset, such as a "thunderclap" headache.
- Change in the nature of a headache, including increased frequency, worsening severity, or new associated symptoms.
- A new headache in a patient with cancer or HIV.
- New-onset headache in a patient more than 50-year old.
- Headache associated with seizures.
- An abnormal neurologic examination including focal deficits or altered mental status.

> KEY FACT | The classic triad of fever, neck stiffness, and altered mental status occurs in only 44% of cases of meningitis.

Regarding meningitis, it's worth pondering a 2004 Dutch study by van de Beek and colleagues [4]. In reviewing almost 700 cases of community-acquired bacterial meningitis, they found that the classic triad of fever, neck stiffness, and a change in mental status was relatively rare, occurring in only 44% of cases. On the other hand, at least two of four signs – fever, neck stiffness, change in mental status, and headache – occurred in 95% of cases; 4% of cases had only one of these symptoms, and 1% none.

Pitfall | Waiting for results before treating suspected bacterial meningitis

> KEY FACT | In cases of suspected meningitis, antibiotics should be administered as soon as possible and should not be delayed pending results from diagnostic studies.

In medicine, order is greatly emphasized. The clinician gathers information, develops a differential, conducts tests, makes a diagnosis, then treats. In EM we frequently challenge this doctrine and when faced with central nervous system (CNS) infections, it is imperative to do so. Two independent, retrospective studies demonstrated that delays in antibiotic therapy increased adverse outcomes and death in the setting of bacterial meningitis [5, 6]. In the case of suspected meningitis, this delay can be deadly, especially when the time to antibiotics exceeds 6 h. The risk imparted by the delay carries more risk than the potential adverse reaction from a single dose of antibiotics. The algorithm, therefore, is antibiotics, then CT and LP. This holds true even when hospital transfer is required to obtain the CT.

The argument that antibiotics will render the cerebrospinal fluid (CSF) non-diagnostic is also unfounded. Initial antibiotic therapy does not change CSF cell counts or protein or glucose. Gram stain and culture may also remain positive despite antibiotic administration. Blood cultures, drawn prior to antibiotic administration, may also reflect the responsible bacterial agent [6, 7].

> KEY FACT | Corticosteroids administered prior to antibiotics may improve outcomes in patients with meningitis.

The 2002 study by de Gans and colleagues added another wrinkle to this series of actions [8]. It demonstrated the importance of not only timely antibiotic therapy, but also timely and coordinated provision of corticosteroids in treating adult bacterial meningitis. In this study of 301 adult patients with meningitis, dexamethasone 10 mg intravenously 15 min prior to antibiotic therapy substantially improved response to therapy, reducing both unfavorable outcomes and death. For patients with suspected meningitis who meet the inclusion criteria of the study – suspicion of meningitis but no cerebrospinal shunt, no pregnancy, no recent antibiotic

therapy, no active tuberculosis or fungal infection, and no recent head trauma, neurosurgery, or peptic ulcer disease – both dexamethasone and antibiotics should be given prior to the diagnostic procedures. Because the theoretical mechanism for the steroid's efficacy is to prevent immunologic response to lysed bacterial proteins, the dexamethasone should be given before or, at the latest, with the antibiotics [9]. If the patient proves not to have meningitis, the therapy can be discontinued, otherwise, it should be continued for 4 days.

Pitfall | Failing to recognize the limitations of a non-contrast head CT

By the time we've completed our discussion of pitfall number 1, and we've all looked for red flags in the diagnosis and treatment of headache (Table 5.2), we are ordering non-contrast CTs on a large percentage of people who enter our departments with headaches. This is not surprising, as the technology is available and common. But it can be deceptively comforting, too, as not all diagnoses will be made on the non-contrast CT. It is for this reason that magnetic resonance imaging (MRI) has become the most desirable test for headache, though it is not as readily available in EM. Even the standard argument that CT scanning is to look for bleed and the MRI for everything else may be falling by the wayside. MRI may be equally as accurate as CT in seeking out acute intracerebral hemorrhage [10].

What might be missed on the non-contrast CT? The list is long, but falls into a few specific categories: vascular disease, neoplastic disease, posterior and cervicomedullary lesions, and infections [11]. As we seek to uncover the odd causes of concerning headaches, therefore, we try to bear in mind that aneurysms themselves will not be visualized on CT, nor will arterial dissections, venous thromboses, early infarctions, or vasculitides. Neoplasms can hide on a non-contrast scan, as can brain abscesses. Posterior lesions and infarctions will hide amidst the scatter of the posterior skull. Pituitary lesions may not be well visualized on the non-contrast CT.

Until we all have MRI available 24 hours daily, it will be beneficial to recall when CT scanning with contrast might be beneficial, improving on the sensitivity of the non-contrast scan. There are, as always, downsides to this approach. There are the risks of renal injury from contrast, along with the risks of contrast reaction, and unintentional injection of contrast into the subcutaneous tissue. The advantage of contrast lies in its ability to show where the blood–brain barrier has broken down. The normal, healthy areas of the barrier will not demonstrate uptake of contrast [12]. Therefore, tumors and inflammatory processes enhance. For the patient with HIV, or in whom metastatic disease is suspected, contrast may be particularly helpful.

In the patient with the worst headache ever, the "thunderclap" headache, or the headache with nuchal rigidity, we often ponder whether to head all the way down the path of the CT and LP. A year 2000 review found three basic categories of reasons for failure to diagnose a subarachnoid hemorrhage: failure to appreciate the spectrum of presentations, failure to understand the limitations of head CT, and failure to perform and interpret a LP [2]. To make matters more complicated, a 2003 review of 90 studies suggested that the only 10–43% of patients with subarachnoid hemorrhage reported a prior "sentinel headache [13]." In other words, the sudden, severe headache, on its own, is not a sensitive indicator for subarachnoid hemorrhage.

> KEY FACT | **The sensitivity of CT to identify subarachnoid hemorrhage decreases with time.**

The limited sensitivity of CT for subarachnoid hemorrhage continues to be a matter of debate as our technology improves. Equally important, though, is recognizing that the sensitivities of the test varies with time. Within 12 h of a subarachnoid hemorrhage, a third-generation CT may identify up to 100% of bleeds. After 12 h however, the sensitivity may fall to 82%, and then continue to fall with time [2, 14]. On the other hand, CT scanners themselves improve with each generation of machines. At least one study suggests that with the advent of new generations of scanners, the LP will eventually become unnecessary in the effort to rule out subarachnoid hemorrhage [15]. Until this is demonstrated consistently, however, a negative CT should never be used in isolation to rule out subarachnoid hemorrhage.

Pitfall | **Trusting the laboratory evaluation of xanthochromia**

Like the CT, CSF analysis is also time dependent. Hemoglobin metabolizes to pink oxyhemoglobin and yellow bilirubin, the colors that make CSF "xanthochromic." Development of the discoloration, though, can take up to 12 h. A traumatic LP may lead to a falsely positive finding of xanthochromia, though more often, it will result in the presence of erythrocytes in the CSF [16].

> KEY FACT | **Visual inspection of CSF for xanthochromia can miss up to 50% of cases.**

Ideally, the hospital laboratory will evaluate CSF with the use of spectrophotometry. Few hospitals, though, actually have appropriate equipment for this [17]. Visual evaluation is much less reliable. This is a small point, but a vital one. If your hospital is not using spectrophotometry, the laboratory technician's estimation of "yellowing" of the spinal fluid is no different from your own. Simply hold the test tube up to the light. Unfortunately, visual inspection can miss xanthochromia up to 50% of the time [2].

Pitfall | **Neglecting those sources of headache that lie outside the skull**

Not all serious headaches derive from intracranial pathology. Unfortunately, "exogenous" causes of headache can be difficult to recall and may present atypically. It is critical to consider these to avoid significant morbidity.

> KEY FACT | **Elderly patients with atypical headaches should have an erythrocyte sedimentation rate checked and steroids should strongly be considered for those with values greater than 50.**

Temporal Arteritis

Headache is the single most common symptom of temporal arteritis. Failure to diagnose and treat may result in permanent vision loss [18]. Almost all sufferers of temporal arteritis are aged 50 or older. The majority are women and the disease is more common among whites than African Americans. While headache is the most common complaint, it is not necessarily a temporal headache. The most helpful corroborating features are jaw claudication and diplopia. Temporal artery findings – including a prominent, tender, or pulseless temporal artery – are the most helpful physical examination findings. Any elderly headache sufferer should be considered at risk for temporal arteritis and suspicion should lead one to obtain an erythrocyte sedimentation rate (ESR). There is no clear cut-off for what level of ESR necessitates therapy, but a value less than 50 is reassuring and makes the disease unlikely. A value greater than 50 should prompt consideration of steroid treatment and urgent temporal artery biopsy.

Acute Angle-Closure Glaucoma

Typically, glaucoma occurs quietly and painlessly, but acute angle-closure glaucoma represents 10% of cases and may present with a chief complaint of headache [19]. It appears more commonly in women, elderly patients, Asians, and those with a family history. Typically patients will have symptoms other than headache alone, potentially including ocular pain and redness, blurred vision, halos around lights, and vomiting. Physical examination may reveal a red eye and a hazy cornea. Any suspicion for the disease should prompt evaluation of intra-ocular pressure.

> KEY FACT | **Clusters of headaches in individuals with a common exposure should prompt consideration of carbon monoxide poisoning.**

Carbon Monoxide Poisoning

Headache is the most common presenting symptom among patients with carbon monoxide poisoning [20]. Unfortunately, other acute effects of carbon monoxide poisoning are diffuse and non-specific. They include nausea, vomiting, weakness, dizziness, blurred vision, and confusion. The nature of the headache itself offers little suggestion of the diagnosis, as the headache associated with carbon monoxide poisoning has few consistent or specific characteristics [21]. With such vague symptoms, it is the history that must drive suspicion. Presentation in the early winter with newly introduced heating systems, new appliances, or multiple family members with similar presentations should prompt consideration of the diagnosis and direct one toward obtaining a carboxyhemoglobin level and having carbon monoxide levels checked in the area of potential exposure.

Pre-eclampsia

The pregnant patient presenting with a headache deserves special consideration for the possibility of pre-eclampsia [22]. The maternal complications of pre-eclampsia are extensive and may include abruption placentae, renal failure, liver failure, preterm delivery, and development of the HELLP syndrome or eclampsia. The complaint of headache in a pregnant patient over 20-week gestation warrants extra attention to blood pressure measurement. If there is any question, patients should be evaluated for proteinuria, elevated liver function tests, and thrombolysis. While the physical symptoms of pre-eclampsia can include blurred vision, epigastric pain, right upper quadrant pain, and mental status changes, headache may be the earliest and most frequent presenting complaint [23].

Table 5.2 Headaches for the EP to find and treat.

Threatening headaches that respond to specific therapies

- Subarachnoid hemorrhage
- Meningitis
- Encephalitis
- Cervico–cranial–artery dissection
- Temporal arteritis
- Acute angle-closure glaucoma
- Hypertensive emergency
- Carbon monoxide poisoning
- Pseudotumor cerebri
- Cerebral venous and dural sinus thrombosis
- Acute stroke: either hemorrhagic or ischemic
- Mass lesions including tumor, abscess, and hematoma

Pitfall | **Neglecting a few odd sources of headache that dwell inside the skull**

A few unusual causes of headache remain among those discussed so far.

Pseudotumor Cerebri

The classic patient with pseudotumor cerebri is an overweight female between 15 and 44 who presents most typically with a daily, retro-ocular headache that is made worse with eye movement. Nausea, vomiting, photophobia, neck, and back pain, diplopia, and visual loss may also be associated with the disorder. Physical examination findings may include pipilledema and visual field constriction. The diagnosis, though, is confirmed via LP by the finding of an intracranial pressure >250 mm of water. Treatment—with volume CSF removal, carbonic anhydrase inhibitors, other diuretics, and short-term corticosteroids – may prevent permanent visual loss [24].

Cerebral Venous Thrombosis

Cerebral venous thrombosis presents with severe headache in more than 90% of patients [25]. Focal neurologic signs and seizures appear in approximately half of patients. The presentation, however, is highly variable and – the challenge for us – the CT scan can be entirely normal. CT venography, if available, may be helpful. The patient at risk – and for whom the diagnosis should be considered – is young or middle aged with unusual headache or stroke-like symptoms. Risk factors include recent head injury, delivery, and oral contraceptive use. Treatments for the condition, including anti-coagulation and control of intracranial hypertension, remain unproven.

Viral Encephalitis

Typical features of a viral encephalitis include headache, fever, seizures, and focal neurologic signs [26]. The responsible viruses may include Herpes viruses, adenoviruses, influenza viruses, and multiple others. In ED decision-making, if headache and fever are severe enough to warrant LP for bacterial meningitis, consideration should be given to empiric coverage with acyclovir for the possibility of a herpes encephalitis, as untreated this disease carries a mortality rate of over 70%.

Pitfall | **Failure to pursue immediate neurosurgical intervention**

It's 2 a.m. An 18-year-old male appears on your doorstep. He is unresponsive. His brother says, he sat down on the stoop, yelled, "I have a headache," and collapsed. His CT shows an acute intra cerebral hemorrhage. Identifying the types of hemorrhage that require neurosurgical intervention is crucial to optimizing outcomes.

It's not always clear what intracerebral hemorrhages benefit from surgical therapy and which do not. Even in the neurosurgical literature, there is considerable debate regarding which cases would benefit from acute intervention. Comparative trials date back to the 1960s [27].

For hemorrhage that is neither aneurysmal nor caused by arteriovenous malformation, it is important to determine the size and location of the bleed. In some settings, immediate and aggressive medical care may be the most beneficial approach, especially for patients with only mild disability. For patients with large hematomas, there may be some survival benefit to hematoma evacuation. For the patient with a mid-size bleed and mid-level functional disability, the decision to evacuate will depend on timing, location of bleed, and neurosurgical opinion. Consider surgical evacuation in young patients with moderate or large lobar hemorrhages associated with clinical deterioration and in patients with basal ganglionic hemorrhages with larger volume, expanding volume, or progressive neurologic deterioration [28].

> KEY FACT | **Patients with infratentorial or cerebellar hemorrhages require emergent neurosurgical consultation for hematoma evacuation.**

Infratentorial, or cerebellar bleeds, offer a much simpler perspective. Even small bleeds can progress rapidly, but the cerebellum can be approached with reduced risk of injury to other cortical structure. Generally any cerebellar bleed with a diameter >3 cm is a candidate for surgical evacuation [28].

The indications for surgery in the case of a ruptured aneurysm are complicated and depend on neurological state of the patient and age. The key in this population is to make the diagnosis of aneurysmal bleeding, as the patient with significant aneurysmal bleeding may benefit from rapid surgical intervention where an equally devastated patient with a non-aneurysmal intracerebral hemorrhage might not [29].

Pitfall | **Not responding fully to the medical management of intracerebral hemorrhage while arranging for neurosurgical evaluation**

The effort to obtain neurosurgical consultation and determination of operability can divert one's attention from the intensive medical therapy that may, ultimately, be more beneficial. The goal of medical therapy is to control intracranial pressure and maintain hemodynamic stability while preventing further bleeding from elevated blood pressure. The most common means of controlling intracranial pressure (ICP) is through control of its proxy, arterial blood pressure. Unfortunately, with impaired autoregulation, arterial blood pressure gives an inaccurate assessment of ICP [28]. There is no clear answer as to what might be the "right" level of blood pressure control, though there is some suggestion that a mean arterial pressure >130 mHg should be controlled [30]. Labetalol and esmolol are appropriate agents for this. Hypotension should also be avoided, with systolic blood pressure kept above 90.

Intubation is warranted for patients who have lost their airway reflexes. Avoid aggressive hyperventilation; the pCO_2 should stay above 28 mmHg to avoid excessive cerebral vasoconstriction. Mannitol is appropriate in the setting of impending or completed herniation. In this setting, the head of the bed should be elevated to 30 degrees. Anticonvulsants reduce the risk of convulsive status epilepticus. Seizing patients should receive benzodiazepines and subsequent phenytoin, valproic acid, or phenobarbital.

Corticosteroids have been used in both subarachnoid hemorrhage and intracerebral hemorrhage in order to reduce swelling in the area of the bleed. There appears, however, to be little evidence to either support or condemn this approach [31]. There may be benefit to treatment with Recombinant Activated Factor VIIA [32]. In any event, anti-coagulation should be reversed in patients on warfarin.

Pitfall | **Attributing headache to elevated blood pressure**

You need only read this particular pitfall if you are familiar with this chief complaint from triage: "I always get a headache when my blood pressure is up. I'd like you to check my blood pressure." Is there any validity to this complaint?

While a 2004 abstract suggests that there might be an association between blood pressure and daily headache in a large screened population in Romania [33], this does not appear to be the case in a large study in a US emergency department. A Philadelphia study evaluating 551 patients found no relationship between blood pressure and symptoms, including headache [34]. A Norwegian study found an inverse relationship between headache and hypertension [35].

A circular argument develops easily in these situations: is the elevated blood pressure causing the headache, or is the pain of the headache leading to an elevated blood pressure? In either case, presuming that a patient's headache arose purely because of underlying hypertension – and is therefore benign – is a dangerous approach.

Pitfall | **Failure to consider a broad armamentarium in the treatment of headache**

> KEY FACT | **Treatment of headache pain should be individualized to the inciting cause.**

Multiple therapies, specific and general, exist for the treatment of headache pain. Many medications have demonstrated efficacy, even though not specifically designed for headache. Fortunately, EPs frequently seem to take advantage of the many options [36]. A review of the 1998 US based National Hospital Ambulatory Medical Care Survey revealed over two-dozen oral and parenteral agents used to treat both migraine and unspecified headache [37]. Common oral medications included acetaminophen, NSAIDS (most commonly ibuprofen and naproxen), and combination medications including hydrocodone/acetaminophen and oxycodone/acetaminophen. Less common medications included tramadol, zolmitriptan, and prednisone. The most common parenteral agents included the parenteral NSAID ketorolac, and parenteral prochlorperazine, metoclopramide, and chlorpromazine. Almost one-third of non-specific headache sufferers received opioid therapy. Use of anti-emetics was common, though mostly in combination with opioid therapy.

The anti-emetics, NSAIDS, and opiates all provide non-specific headache therapy. Each delivers its own side effects, as well. The anti-emetics, prochlorperazine, and promethazine, carry the risk of extrapyramidal symptoms, most notably a dystonia and akathisia. These symptoms reverse with diphenhydramine. Droperidol, another non-specific headache treatment, though not alone in causing QT interval prolongation, has earned a special warning in the US for this side effect. The NSAIDS risk gastrointestinal upset and, in long-term use, bleeding, and many patients have already tried them at home. The opiates tend to sedate patients, prevent them from safely driving home and carry with them the potential for dependence.

Some headaches suggest specific, individualized therapy. Migraine headaches, for example, have their own armamentarium [38]. The specific pharmacologic migraine treatments include the ergotamines and triptans, though many migraine sufferers will have already tried one of these prior to coming to the ED. With their mechanism of vasoconstriction, these medications are somewhat limited and even dangerous as a diagnostic tool and are probably best avoided in the undefined headache. A 2005 meta-analysis suggests that dihydroergotamine is less effective than sumatriptan or phenothiazines as a single agent – suggesting the value of starting therapy, even for migraines, with a phenothiazine or anti-emetic [39]. In the same meta-analysis, however, combined treatment with dihydroergotamine and an anti-emetic – typically metoclopramide – outperformed treatment with meperidine, valproate, or ketorolac. The long-term non-pharmacologic therapies for migraine – exercise, sleep, regular diet, avoidance of dietary triggers – are all tactics of which we may remind patients, but for which the diligence of daily compliance relies much more on regular primary and neurologic care.

Additional alternative remedies may be appropriate in a number of settings. Oxygen effectively treats cluster headaches. Injection of local anesthetic at occipital and temporal locations where applied pressure increases symptoms may relieve recalcitrant headaches [40]. If muscle strain and torticollis are the underlying cause, muscle relaxants may be helpful. There is some evidence that acupuncture may be a useful treatment for idiopathic headache [41].

Pearls for Improving Patient Outcomes

- Consider a more extensive search for serious pathology in patients with headache who are elderly, immunosuppressed, have abnormal neurologic findinigs, or have a headache which is atypical of their usual pattern of headache pain.
- Do not rely on the presence of the "classic" triad of fever, neck stiffness, and altered mental status to consider the diagnosis of meningitis.
- When meningitis is suspected, antibiotics should be administered immediately while waiting for diagnostic test results.
- CT cannot be used in isolation to rule out subarachnoid hemorrhage.
- CSF should be analyzed spectophotometrically to assess for xanthochromia to maximize diagnostic yield.
- Temporal arteritis, acute angle-closure glaucoma, pre-eclampsia, and carbon monoxide poisoning must be considered in at risk patients.
- Infratentorial and cerebellar hematomas must prompt emergent neurosurgical consultation.
- Pharmacologic treatment of headache pain should be tailored to the likely etiology.

References

1. Raskin NH. Headache. In: Kasper DL, et al. (eds), *Harrison's Principles of Internal Medicine*, 16th ed. New York: McGraw-Hill, 2005, pp. 85–94.
2. Edlow JA, Caplan LR. Avoiding pitfalls in the diagnosis of subarachnoid hemorrhage. *New Engl J Med* 2000; 342:29–36.
3. American College of Emergency Physicians. Clinical Policy: critical issues in the evaluation and management of patients presenting to the emergency department with acute headache. *Ann Emerg Med* 2002; 39:108–22.
4. Van de Beek D, de Gans J, Spanjaard L, Weisfelt M, Reitsma JB, Vermeulen M. Clinical features and prognostic factors in adults with bacterial meningitis. *New Engl J Med* 2004; 351:1849–59.
5. Aronin SI, Peduzzi P, Quagliarello VJ. Community-acquired bacterial meningitis: risk stratification for adverse clinical outcome and effect of antibiotic timing. *Ann Intern Med* 1998; 129:862–9.
6. Proulx N, Frechette D, Toye B, Chan J, Kravcik S. Delays in the administration of antibiotics are associated with mortality from adult acute bacterial meningitis. *QJM* 2005; 98:291–8.
7. Talan DA, Hoffman JR, Yoshikawa TT, Overturf GD. Role of empiric antibiotics prior to lumbar puncture in suspected bacterial meningitis: state of the art. *Rev Infect Dis* 1988; 10:365–76.
8. deGans J, Van de Beek D. Dexamethasone in adults with bacterial meningitis. *New Engl J Med* 2002; 347:1549–56.
9. Van de Beek D, de Gans J, Tunkel AR, Wijdicks EFM. Community-acquired bacterial meningitis in adults. *New Engl J Med* 2006; 354:44–53.
10. Kidwell CS, Chalela JA, Saver JL, et al. Comparison of MRI and CT for detection of acute intracerebral hemorrhage. *J Am Med Assoc* 2004; 292:1823–30.
11. Silberstein SD, Lipton RB, Goadsby PJ. Diagnostic testing and ominous causes of headache. In: Silberstein SD, Lipton RB, Goadsby PJ (eds), *Headache in Clinical Practice*, 2nd edn. London: Martin Dunitz Ltd, 2002, pp. 35–46.
12. Sklar EM, Ruiz A, Quencer RM, Falcone SF Structural neuroimaging. In: Bradley WG, Daroff RB, Fenichel GM, Jankovic J (eds), *Neurology in Clinical Practice: Principles of Diagnosis and Management*, 4th ed. Philadelphia: Butterworth Heinemann, 2004, pp. 521–97.

13. Polmear A. Sentinel headaches in aneurismal subarachnoid haemorrhage: what is the true incidence? A systematic review. *Cephalgia* 2003; 23:935–41.

14. Sidman R, Connolly E, Lemke T. Subarachnoid hemorrhage diagnosis: lumbar puncture is still needed when the computed tomography scan is normal. *Acad Emerg Med* 1996; 3:827–31.

15. Boesiger BM, Shiber JR. Subarachnoid hemorrhage diagnosis by computed tomography and lumbar puncture: are fifth generation CT scanners better at identifying subarachnoid hemorrhage? *J Emerg Med* 2005; 29(1):23–27.

16. Graves P, Sidman R. Xanthochromia is not pathognomonic for subarachnoid hemorrhage. *Acad Emerg Med* 2004; 11(2):131–35.

17. Edlow JA, Bruner KS, Horowitz GL. Xanthochromia: a survey of laboratory methodology and its clinical implications. *Arch Pathol Lab Med* 2002; 126:413–15.

18. Smetana GW, Schmerling RH. Does this patient have temporal arteritis? *J Am Med Assoc* 2002; 287:92–101.

19. Lee DA, Higginbotham EJ. Glaucoma and its treatment: a review. *Am J Health-Syst Pharm* 2005; 62:691–99.

20. Kao LW, Nañagas HA. Carbon monoxide poisoning. *Med Clin N Am* 2005; 89:1161–94.

21. Hampson NB, Hampson LA. Characteristics of headache associated with acute carbon monoxide poisoning. *Headache* 2002; 42:220–23.

22. Sibai B, Dekker G, Kupferminc M. Pre-eclampsia. *Lancet* 2005; 365:785–99.

23. Sibai BM. Diagnosis, prevention, and management of eclampsia. *Obstet & Gynecol* 2005; 105:402–10.

24. Friedman DI. Pseudotumor cerebri. *Neurol Clin N Am* 2004; 22:99–131.

25. Stam J. Thrombosis of the cerebral veins and sinuses. *New Engl J Med* 2005; 352(17):1791–98.

26. Kennedy PGE. Viral encephalitis. *J Neurol* 2005; 252:268–72.

27. Singh RVP, Prusmack CJ, Morcos JJ. Spontaneous intracerebral hemorrhage: non-arteriovenous malformation, nonaneurysm. In: Winn HR (ed). *Youmans Neurological Surgery*, 5th ed. Philadelphia: Saunders, 2004, pp. 1733–68.

28. Qureshi AI, Tuhrim S, Broderick JP, Batjer HH, Hondo H, Hanley DF. Spontaneous intracerebral hemorrhage. *New Engl J Med* 2001; 344:1450–60.

29. Roux PDL, Winn HR. Surgical decision making for the treatment of cerebral aneurysms. In: Winn HR (ed). *Youmans Neurological Surgery*, 5th ed. Philadelphia: Saunders, 2004, pp. 1793–1812.

30. Mayer SA, Rincon F. Treatment of intracerebral haemorrhage. *Lancet Neurol* 2005; 4:662–72.

31. Feigin VL, Anderson N, Rikel GJE, Algra A, van Gijn J, Bennett DA. Corticosteroids for aneurysmal subarachnoid haemorrhage and primary intracerebral haemorrhage. *The Cochrane Database of Systematic Reviews* 2005; 3: CD004583.

32. Juvela S, Kase C. Advances in intracerebral hemorrhage management. *Stroke* 2006; 37(2):301–04.

33. Gordon PE, Chiang WK, Hexdall WK, Kovacs M, Levy P, Compton S, Arafat R. Headache and hypertension – is there an association? [Abstract] *Acad Em Med* 2004; 11(5)521.

34. Karras DJ, Ufberg JW, Harrigan RA, Wald DA, Botros MS, McNamara RM. Lack of relationship between hypertension-associated symptoms and blood pressure in hypertensive ED patients. *Am J Emerg Med* 2005; 23:106–10.

35. Hagen K, Stovner LJ, Vatten L, et al. Blood pressure and risk of headache: a prospective study of 22,685 adults in Norway. *J Neurol Neurosurg Psychiatry* 2002; 72:463–66.

36. Vinson DR, Hurtado TR, Vandenberg JT, Banwart L. Variations among emergency departments in the treatment of benign headache. *Ann Emerg Med* 2003; 41:90–97.

37. Vinson DR. Treatment patterns of isolated benign headache in US emergency departments. *Ann Emerg Med* 2002; 39:215–22.

38. Goadsby PJ, Lipton RB, Ferrari MD. Migraine – current understanding and treatment. *New Engl J Med* 2002; 346:257–70.

39. Colman I, Brown MD, Innes GD, Grafstein E, Roberts TE, Rowe BH. Parenteral dihydroergotamine for acute migraine headache: a systematic review of the literature. *Ann Emerg Med* 2005; 45: 393–401.

40. Brofeldt BT, Panacek EA. Pericranial injection of local anesthetics for the management of resistant headaches. *Acad Emerg Med* 1998; 5:1224–29.

41. Melchart D, Linde K, Berman B, White A, Vickers A, Allais G, Brinkhaus B. Acupuncture for idiopathic headache. *The Cochrane Database of Systematic Reviews* 2001; 1: CD001218.

Chapter 6 | **Evaluation and Management of the Patient with Neck Pain**

Joshua Broder & Anita L'Italien

Introduction

Neck pain can be a daunting problem in the emergency department, with etiologies ranging from benign to life threatening. The neck contains vascular, nerve, airway, digestive, and bony structures, any of which may be the source of pain. In addition, referred pain from other regions of the body may present with neck pain. Fascial planes connect compartments of the neck with the mediastinum and prevertebral spaces, posing a risk of spread of infection from the neck to these regions. Pitfalls in the management of the patient with neck pain include failure to consider the diverse differential diagnosis, diagnostic failures due to reliance on insensitive features of the history and exam, misunderstanding of the limitations of diagnostic laboratory and imaging tests, and failure to treat with specific therapy in a timely fashion. In this chapter we'll consider some unusual but dangerous causes of neck pain which are prone to pitfalls in diagnosis and treatment, including infections, vascular disasters, and spinal cord compression syndromes. Pitfalls in the diagnosis and treatment of cervical spine trauma are discussed separately in the chapter pertaining to the trauma.

Pitfall | **Failure to consider a vascular cause of neck pain**

> KEY FACT | **Internal carotid artery dissection is the most common cause of stroke in young adults.**

Cervical artery dissection (CAD) is a rare condition. Failure to recognize it can lead to subsequent devastating neurologic impairment from ischemic or thrombotic events. Unlike aortic dissection, CAD is a disease predominantly of the young with 70% occurring in people aged 20–40 years [1]. Internal carotid artery dissection (ICAD) is the most common cause of stroke in young adults. Headache and neck pain are prominent features and up to 25% of people experience neck pain alone [1, 2]. Isolated neck pain is more common in ICAD than in vertebral artery dissection (VAD). The neck pain of CAD is usually sudden, severe, and persistent pain.

CAD occurs after major blunt trauma, but also after trivial trauma such as coughing, defecation, sexual activity, sporting activities, and chiropractic manipulation. One study found that 16% of CAD occurred after chiropractic treatments [3]. Apparently spontaneous dissections are also well documented in the literature [3–10]. Other risk factors include history of migraines, hypertension, tobacco use, connective tissue disorders, and vasculitides.

Pitfall | **Reliance on a normal physical exam to rule out arterial dissection**

The most common presentation of ICAD is headache and/or neck pain with ischemic symptoms that may not present until several hours or even days after the onset of neck pain. 36–58% of patients will have an incomplete Horner's syndrome (ptosis and miosis without anhydrosis) and <15% will have lower cranial nerve palsies [1]. In addition to headache or neck pain, VAD presents with posterior circulation stroke or cerebellar signs such as vertigo (57%), nausea/vomiting (53%), unilateral facial numbness (46%), unsteadiness/gait disturbance (42%), diplopia (23%), dysarthria (15%), dysphagia (11%), or extremity paresthesias or weakness (11%) [2]. Symptoms can be transient and neurological deficits can be subtle or absent at presentation.

When CAD is suspected based on history or physical examination, radiologic imaging should be obtained to rule in or rule out the diagnosis. Helical computed tomographic (CT) cervical angiography is the diagnostic test of choice for CAD in the emergency department due to its excellent sensitivity and specificity (both approaching 100%), availability and rapidity of testing, ability to evaluate several alternative diagnoses, and the non-invasive nature of the test (see Figure 6.1). Alternative diagnostic techniques include conventional cervical angiography (78–84% sensitive), vascular ultrasound, or MRI/MRA of the head and neck which is >95% sensitive. As with any testing technique, false positive and false negative results may rarely occur with CT angiography, sometimes for technical reasons such as metallic streak artifacts in the image field or failure to include the entire artery in question. If significant suspicion for this diagnosis exists despite a normal diagnostic imaging exam, an additional exam using a different test modality should be considered [11].

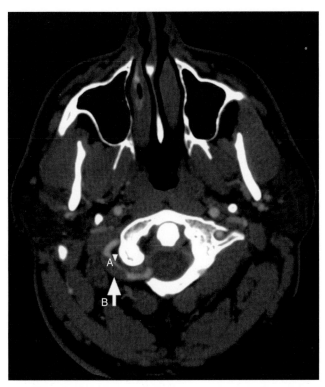

Figure 6.1 VAD on CT with IV contrast.
The patient's right vertebral artery shows a stenotic region (arrow A), with near complete loss of the lumen at the level of the C2 ring in the extraforaminal portion of the vessel. The dark gray region (arrow B) is a thrombosed region of dissection.

> KEY FACT | **CAD should be considered in any adult patient complaining of sudden onset of significant neck pain with a history of trauma, however minor, or recent chiropractic manipulation.**

CAD should be considered in any adult patient complaining of a sudden onset of significant neck pain with a history of trauma, however minor, or recent chiropractic manipulation. Ischemic symptoms, visual changes and symptoms of posterior stroke should be sought in the history. A thorough neurological examination, especially of the cranial nerves, is essential. A normal neurological exam in a patient with a suspicious history does not rule out the diagnosis and should prompt radiologic testing.

Pitfall | **Failure to consider a cardiac cause of neck pain**

Neck pain is a well-known manifestation of cardiac ischemia, although usually as an additional feature of classical anginal symptoms such as chest pain or dyspnea. Rare case reports describe patients with cervical pain as the sole expression of coronary artery disease, although often in retrospect more

typical features of cardiac chest pain are evident, though subtle [12]. The presence of arm pain associated with neck pain may be interpreted as radiculopathy when in fact both symptoms are related to coronary ischemia. Unfortunately, symptoms of either radiculopathy or angina pectoris can be exacerbated by ambulation, position, or arm motions, confounding the diagnosis. Consideration of a cardiac cause of neck pain should be given in patients with multiple cardiac risk factors, no history of trauma, and particularly when diagnostic evaluations for cervical pathology have been negative. A careful review of associated symptoms should be performed. Women may be more likely than men to describe neck pain as a symptom of cardiac ischemia [13].

Pitfall | **Failure to recognize an infectious cause of neck pain**

Physicians may fail to recognize an infectious cause of neck pain for a variety of reasons, including incomplete differential diagnosis or over-reliance on specific history, exam, laboratory, and imaging data. Treatment failures may also occur, including failure to administer antibiotics or failure to involve a surgical consultant.

> KEY FACT | **Deep cervical infections may spread via fascial planes to the mediastinum, resulting in mediastinitus with a mortality as high as 60%.**

A variety of significant infections within the neck may present with neck pain (see Table 6.1). These include peritonsillar, parapharyngeal, and retropharyngeal abscesses, epiglottitis, Ludwig's angina, meningitis, osteomyelitis, diskitis, cervical epidural abscesses (CEA), mastoiditis, otitis, and dental infections. Infections of congenital structures such as branchial cleft cysts and thyroglossal duct cysts may occur. Some unusual forms of pharyngitis may cause severe neck or throat pain, including diphtheria, and esophagitis from herpes, CMV (cytomegalovirus), or candida infection. Lemierre's syndrome, an infectious thrombophlebitis of the internal jugular venous system, can be devastating and may present with neck pain. Deep cervical plane infections may spread via fascial planes to the mediastinum, resulting in mediastinitis with a mortality as high as 60% [14].

> KEY FACT | **In the vaccine era, adult cases of acute epiglottitis outnumber pediatric cases.**

Epiglottitis has seen a decline in children since the introduction of the Hib vaccine in the early 1990s. However, the disease continues to be found in *adults* at rates similar to or higher than in the pre-vaccine era [15, 16]. In fact, in the vaccine era, adult cases of acute epiglottitis (83%) outnumber

Table 6.1 Infectious causes of neck pain.

Peritonsillar abscess
Parapharyngeal abscess
Retropharyngeal abscess
Epiglottitis
Ludwig's angina
Meningitis
Osteomyelitis
Diskitis
Cervical epidural abscess
Mastoiditis
Otitis
Dental infections
Infections of congenital structures (e.g. branchial cleft cysts,
  thyroglossal duct cysts)
Pharyngitis
Esophagitis
Lemierre's syndrome
Deep cervical plane infections

pediatric cases (17%) [17]. In addition, although rare, *Haemophilus influenza*-related epiglottitis can be found in *fully vaccinated children*. A 10-year retrospective study in New England found 19 cases of childhood epiglottitis in a single children's hospital, 6 positive for *H. influenzae*, and 5 of those 6 in children with up-to-date immunizations [18].

Pitfall | **Failure to elicit historical or exam findings suggesting infection**

A history of injection drug use should prompt consideration of venous thrombosis or deep neck abscesses, including epidural spinal abscess. Retained foreign bodies such as needle fragments may also provide a nidus for infection. In a retrospective review, patients failed to disclose a history of cervical injection in 50% of cases [19, 20]. Cervical osteomyelitis has been reported as a complication of cervical injection [21, 22]. Swallowed foreign bodies such as bone fragments may also cause deep space infection. A history of incomplete immunization or immigrant status may place the patient at risk of diphtheria infection. Immune compromise such as HIV/AIDS should prompt consideration of infection with herpes, CMV, or candida. Neurological complaints may suggest CEA. Recent infections, including distant sources such as UTI or skin abscesses, can lead to deep space infections, meningitis or CEA by hematogenous inoculation.

Patients with a "*locus minoris resistantiae*" of the cervical spine may be at increased risk for hematogenous seeding. Examples include spondylosis, degenerative joint disease, previous laminectomy or non-penetrating trauma from a fall or motor vehicle collision. Some underlying diseases also predispose patients to developing CEAs such as diabetes mellitus, alcoholism, cancer, chronic renal failure and those with compromised immune states. Any previous invasive spinal procedure,

even several months prior to presentation, should increase the suspicion of CEA. Patients typically will not offer this information unless asked specifically; 18% percent of patients will have no identifiable predisposing factors for CEA [23, 24].

Physical exam should be thorough, but normal findings should be incorporated into the overall picture, not used in isolation to exclude a disease entity. Careful attention should be paid to temperature, heart rate, blood pressure, and respiratory rate. The neck should be inspected for asymmetry or swelling. Palpation for fluctuance or adenopathy should be performed. The thyroid should be examined. Any stridor or pooling of secretions should be noted. The oropharynx should be inspected, looking for lesions or swelling. The dentition and sublingual spaces should be examined. The uvula position should be noted, especially any deviation. Tonsils should be examined for swelling or exudates. Trismus and spitting of secretions are also ominous signs. Brawny edema of the submandibular region and elevation of the tongue are signs of Ludwig's angina. A pseudomembrane should prompt consideration of diphtheria. A careful neurological examination of the cranial nerves and upper extremities should be performed if suggested by history or symptoms.

Pitfall | **Reliance on the absence of classic physical exam findings to rule out infection**

The classic physical exam findings of many dangerous neck infections are not reliably present in patients with disease, and their absence should not be used to rule out pathology. Although neck stiffness is a common complaint in meningitis (88%) [25], classic exam signs of meningitis should *not* be relied upon due to poor sensitivity: a prospective study found Kernig's sign and Brudzinski's signs to be only 5% sensitive for meningitis, and nuchal rigidity to be only 30% sensitive [26]. According to a retrospective review comparing physical exam and symptoms with CT diagnosis of deep neck infection, the physical exam for deep cervical infections is relatively insensitive, underestimating the extent of infection in 70% of patients. Classic signs and symptoms of infection were present with the following frequency: fever (75.4%), pain (89.2%), odynophagia (63.1%), dysphagia (47.7%), neck swelling (84.6%), localized pain (76.9%), local erythema (66.7%), and localized increase in temperature (55.4%) [27]. In epiglottitis, drooling is a presenting symptom in only 15.2%, and stridor or dyspnea in only 8.6%. Although "hot potato" voice may suggest epiglottitis [28], muffled voice is found in just over half of patients (52.1%) [29].

Pitfall | **Over-reliance on fever as a sign of infection**

KEY FACT | **In patients with meningitis ... absence of a fever at presentation is associated with nearly 40-fold increased mortality.**

Fever is an unreliable finding. Reviews of presenting symptoms of adult patients with epiglottis found mean presenting temperature to be 37.4°C [28, 29]. In patients with meningitis, fever is sometimes absent (7–33%), and absence of a fever status at presentation is associated with nearly 40-fold increased mortality (odds ratio 39.4), perhaps due to delay in antibiotic administration [30, 31]. In patients with CEA, fever was present in only 79% of patient in one review [23] and was >38.4 in only 32% of patients in another large review [32]. In yet another study, the mean presenting temperature was only 38° C [33]. The classic triad of localized spine tenderness, progressive neurological deficits, and fever occurs in only 37% of patients with CEA [34].

Pitfall | Reliance on peripheral WBC count to exclude infection

Laboratory tests may assist in the diagnosis of infection, but over-reliance on test results such as WBC count may result in misdiagnosis. A review of epiglottis presentations found mean WBC counts of 14,134.4 ± 5556.1/mm^3, meaning that a significant percentage of patients presented with counts within the normal range (5000–10,000/mm^3) [29]. Cases have been reported of epiglottitis with normal WBC counts and no fever [35].

> KEY FACT | In children younger than 90 days, a low WBC count ... is associated with a seven times higher risk of meningitis compared to the risk of bacteremia.

In children younger than 90 days, a low WBC count (less than 5000 cells/mm^3) actually is associated with a seven times higher risk of meningitis compared to the risk of bacteremia [36]. In adults, serum leukocyte count has not been shown to be a useful test to rule out meningitis. Published cohorts of community-acquired meningitis include significant numbers of patients with low, normal, and high peripheral WBC counts [37]. The peripheral WBC count should *not* be used as a decision node to discontinue a workup for meningitis.

In CEA, an elevated WBC count is an unreliable finding as it is normal in up to 40% of patients [32]. 95% of patients will have an elevated erythrocyte sedimentation rate (ESR) with an average value of 51 mm/h but this is also a non-specific finding [32, 38].

WBC counts may not be elevated in the presence of significant infection or abscess, and low or normal WBC counts may occur in acutely infected but immunocompromised hosts.

Pitfall | Misinterpretation of cerebrospinal fluid results

Cerebrospinal fluid (CSF) testing may be misinterpreted to rule out meningitis inappropriately. Among patients with relatively low CSF WBC counts, the presence of markedly abnormal protein, neutrophil, or glucose values increases the

likelihood of bacterial meningitis. Intermediate values of these CSF markers have little diagnostic value. Specifically, in children with CSF WBC less than 30/mm^3, high likelihood ratios for bacterial meningitis are found for protein greater than 120 mg/dl (LR 22), neutrophil count greater than 75% (LR 57), glucose less than 20 mg/dl (LR 15), and glucose greater than 120 mg/dl (LR 20) [39]. The same investigators have reported a formula to discriminate between bacterial and viral meningitis in children with CSF white cell counts greater than 7/mm^3, based on CSF glucose and protein, CSF neutrophil count, and patient age. They report a "high" sensitivity; however, the actual range of sensitivities reported varies between 92% and 98% [40], which may be unacceptable to an individual practitioner. This rule has not been validated, and no similar rule has been used in adults. Other decision rules for discriminating bacterial from viral meningitis in children have been derived and validated. The Bacterial Meningitis Score has been described as a sensitive discriminator between bacterial and viral meningitis. The score (1 point each for CSF protein ≥80 mg/dl, peripheral absolute neutrophil count ≥10,000 cells/mm^3, seizure before or at presentation, and CSF neutrophil count ≥1000 cells/mm^3, and 2 points for a CSF Gram stain showing bacteria) has a reported negative predictive value of 100% when the score is 0, but a sensitivity of only 87% for bacterial meningitis when the score is 2 or more [41].

An additional consideration is the difference between sensitivity and negative predictive value. Sensitivity is the ability of a test to be positive in patients with disease, and it is independent of the prevalence of a disease in a population. In contrast, negative predictive value refers to the likelihood of absence of disease when the test is negative. Negative predictive value is subject to change, depending on the prevalence of disease. In a pediatric study, a CSF WBC count less than 30 cells/mm^3 was associated with a negative predictive value for bacterial meningitis of 99.3%, in a population of 1617 patients undergoing lumbar puncture. While this value seems quite good, in fact only 44 patients (2.7%) had confirmed meningitis, so almost *any* test, even a poor one, could indicate the absence of disease 97.3% of the time. *But* of the 44 cases of bacterial meningitis which were identified, 5 had 0–3 cells/mm^3, and 6 had 4–30 cells/mm^3, giving a cutoff of 30 cells a sensitivity of only 75% [42]!

Correction of the CSF results for suspected traumatic lumbar puncture represents another opportunity for pitfall. Evidence is scant that a corrected CSF value is a valid test for meningitis, with a single published article suggesting that a CSF WBC count greater than 10 times that attributable to trauma is a sensitive cut-off for meningitis [43].

Pitfall | Reliance on plain film to exclude deep neck infection

Classic plain film findings of epiglottitis (see Figure 6.2; see Table 6.2), while helpful if present, may be inadequate to

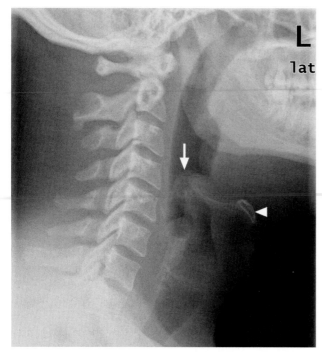

Figure 6.2 Epiglottitis on plain film
This lateral soft tissue neck film demonstrates a classic "thumbprint sign" (arrow) of an inflamed epiglottis. The hyoid bone is also seen (arrowhead). Of note, this is an adult patient, as shown by the mature cervical vertebrae.

Table 6.2 Sensitivities and specificities for plain radiograph findings in epiglottitis

Plain radiograph findings for epiglottitis	Sensitivity (%)	Specificity (%)
Epiglottis width to anterior-posterior (AP) width of C4 >0.33	96	100
Prevertebral soft tissue to C4 ratio >0.5	37	100
Width of hypopharyngeal airway to width of C4 >1.5	44	87
Aryepiglottic fold enlargement	85	100
Arytenoid swelling	70	100

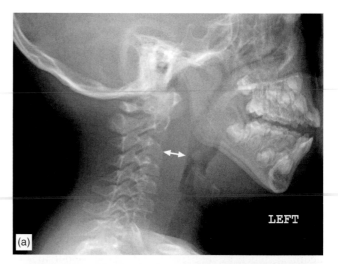

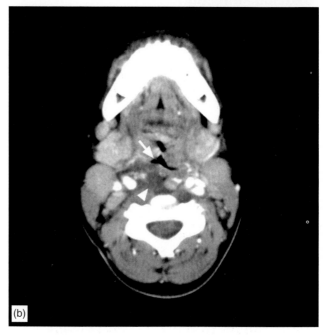

Figure 6.3. Retropharyngeal abscess in a 6-year-old male with sore throat.
(a) Lateral view of the neck shows abnormal widening of the prevertebral soft tissues (double arrow). Although a variety of criteria have been described, soft tissues which exceed the width of the adjacent vertebral bodies should raise suspicion of abscess. (b) CT with IV contrast shows an ill-defined hypoattenuation and soft tissue prominence in the right retropharyngeal space (arrowhead), representing an abscess. The airway (arrow) is displaced anteriorly by the abscess.

rule out the diagnosis [44]. CT may be used to diagnose equivocal cases and to delineate complications such as local abscess formation – of course with careful attention to the patient's airway while at CT [45].

Lateral neck X-ray (see Figure 6.3a) for suspected retropharyngeal abscess has a limited sensitivity, around 80%, while CT (see Figure 6.3b) is extremely sensitive (100%) for soft tissue abnormalities associated with retropharyngeal abscesses and cellulitis [46, 47].

When evaluating for retained foreign body, reliance on plain X-ray is a potential pitfall. Cadaver studies comparing CT and plain film for a variety of fish bones found CT uniformly

superior, with a sensitivity around 90% compared with 39% for X-ray [48, 49].

CT itself may have limitations that restrict its use in the management decision for deep neck infections. In studies comparing the ability of CT to discriminate between cellulitis and abscess, with surgical findings used as the gold standard, CT is between 68% and 73.5% sensitive and 56% specific for abscess [50, 51].

Pitfall | **Delaying treatment of serious infections**

Patients at risk for meningitis or diphtheria should immediately undergo respiratory isolation and begin antibiotic therapy. Delay greater than 6 h in antibiotic therapy for meningitis is associated with a significant increase in mortality, with estimates from nearly 2-fold to perhaps 40-fold. Delay in diagnosis due to CT scan preceding lumbar puncture increases the risk of delay in antibiotic administration by a factor of 5.6.

In the case of CEA, emergent neurosurgical consultation should be obtained after the administration of intravenous antibiotics. Neurological function continues to deteriorate in a significant portion of patients after initiation of antibiotics and many experts believe that surgery is necessary even if no neurological deficits are present on diagnosis. About 50% of patients treated medically and admitted without neurologic deficits will have neurological deficits on discharge compared to 20% of those treated surgically before the development of deficits [52]. Additionally, total paralysis can occur in a matter of a few hours. Once neurological symptoms develop, simple removal of the mass may not result in complete recovery because other processes likely occur, in addition to the mechanical compression, that result in cord ischemia such as venous thrombosis or focal septic emboli. Ultimate outcome is likely determined by a number of factors including the duration of symptoms, the only factor where it is possible for emergency physicians to effect a change (by prompt diagnosis, antibiotic therapy, and consultation with a neurosurgeon). Once paralysis develops, it is usually irreversible if surgery is not performed within 24 h of onset [23]. In a review of 188 patients, treatment initiated after 36 h of weakness or paralysis resulted in complete recovery in only 39% of patients [53].

Pitfall | **Failure to consider a neck mass**

> KEY FACT | In patients above the age of 40 years with solitary, benign-appearing cervical cysts, metastatic squamous cell carcinoma may be found in up to 23.5%.

Neck pain may be due to the presence of a previously undiagnosed cervical mass. These include malignant and benign neoplasms and congenital structures such as branchial cleft cysts or thyroglossal duct cysts, which may be super-infected. Associated symptoms of weight loss, dysphagia or odynophagia, hoarseness, or neurological symptoms such as ptosis may suggest malignancy. Cervical neoplasms increase in incidence with age, although some neoplasms, such as lymphomas, may occur in younger patients. In patients above the age of 40 years with solitary, benign-appearing cervical cysts, metastatic squamous cell carcinoma may be found in up to 23.5% [54]. Cigarette smoking and alcohol use are risk factors [55].

Congenital abnormalities may present with neck pain. These include thyroglossal duct cysts in the midline and branchial cleft cysts in the lateral neck. Both thyroglossal duct cysts and branchial cleft cysts may be occult until infection occurs, presenting then with pain and swelling.

Pitfall | **Failure to evaluate the patient for evidence of malignancy**

The physical exam should include inspection of the oropharynx for lesions, as oral cancers may spread locally or metastasize within the neck. The neck should be inspected for asymmetry, and palpation should be performed, including the thyroid gland and anterior and posterior lymph nodes. The voice quality should be noted, and the patient should be asked about changes in voice character. Although hoarseness may be associated with a benign diagnosis such as laryngitis, hoarseness or change in voice could indicate local involvement of laryngeal structures or involvement of the recurrent laryngeal nerve. A Horner's syndrome (ptosis, miosis, anhidrosis) can occur from compression of sympathetic nerves innervating the face, so the patient's eyes should be examined for eyelid position and pupillary size and reactivity. Unfortunately, characteristics from exam and history, including location, number of lesions, bilaterality, size, and duration, have poor positive and negative predictive values for malignancy, in the range of 60–80% [55].

Pitfall | **Reliance on plain film to exclude a mass**

Due to the insensitivity of history and exam for masses, patients with unexplained neck pain may require imaging for further diagnosis. Plain films of the neck are insensitive and not generally useful. If a mass is considered, enhanced CT (CT with IV contrast) is the preferred test, with excellent sensitivity. MRI is helpful in patients with contraindications to iodinated contrast, and ultrasound plays a role in differentiating solid from cystic masses [56].

Pitfall | **Failure to involve a consultant in patients with mass lesions**

Newly diagnosed cervical neoplasms require prompt follow-up, though admission may not be required if the airway is not threatened, the patient is tolerating oral intake, and pain is adequately controlled. A firm outpatient follow-up plan should be in place, with a clear understanding from the patient of the significance of the emergency department findings and potential diagnosis. Otolaryngology referral is advisable for all cervical masses, even those that appear to be benign or local infections, as malignancy may co-exist. Importantly, incision and drainage of cervical masses should rarely be performed by emergency physicians. Some cervical masses, including thyroglossal duct lesions, require complete excision for cure [57]. Emergency department incision and drainage may also be contraindicated because in rare cases these lesions contain the patient's only functional thyroid tissue. Moreover, incision of an unsuspected malignancy may promote spread and compromise chance for surgical cure, due to seeding of malignant cells in needle tracks [58, 59]. Missed diagnoses of laryngeal malignancy can have devastating medical consequences for patients, with high rates of laryngectomy (63%) and mortality (35%). Patients with misdiagnosed laryngeal carcinoma present at an early age (mean 47 years), compared with the peak incidence of the disease (age 70–74 years). Malpractice awards occur in over half of cases [60].

Pitfall | Failure to consider spinal epidural hematoma in patients with neck pain and upper extremity paresthesias or weakness

Cervical epidural hematomas (CEH) are rare, but life threatening. Mortality is 30% for CEH located above C5 [61]. CEH are almost uniformly fatal secondary to respiratory failure if not corrected [62]. Failure to recognize the diagnosis promptly leads to a less favorable outcome and more severe permanent neurological deficits. Because they are so rare, can occur spontaneously, and present with non-specific symptoms, they present a difficult diagnostic dilemma.

CEHs are caused by trauma, underlying hematological disorders or systemic disease, or as a complication of epidural anesthesia [63]. However, there are many reports of spontaneous spinal epidural hematomas (SSEH) in the literature which are defined as occurring in the absence of one of the above causes [61, 62, 64–69]. They occur in as many as 40–50% of cases. SSEH has been reported to occur after minor physical exertion, sneezing, coitus, straining, vomiting, micturition, coughing and bending over. There are several case reports of CEHs occurring after chiropractic manipulation [70–73]. Other risk factors include anticoagulation, prior thrombolytic therapy, pregnancy, alcoholism, liver disease, and rheumatologic disorders.

Pitfall | Reliance on a normal neurologic exam to exclude spinal epidural hematoma

The usual presentation is that of an acute onset of severe posterior neck pain that progresses to para- or tetraplegia in hours or days. Cervical radicular pain is one of the earliest symptoms and a hallmark of cervical epidural hematoma [74]. Although most neck pain due to trauma that presents with radicular symptoms will be due to an injured cervical disk or nerve root, the emergency physician should consider the diagnosis of SSEH and perform a thorough neurological examination. The presence of other risk factors may necessitate imaging to rule out a hematoma.

Pitfall | Failure to perform timely and appropriate imaging and consultation for spinal epidural hematoma

Diagnosis requires MRI or CT *myelography*, and the diagnosis may be missed on non-contrast CT or CT angiography performed for suspected CAD. Treatment involves emergent decompressive laminectomy with clot evacuation. It is also *imperative* to reverse any existing coagulopathy.

Early neurosurgical involvement is essential. The duration of symptoms affects the outcome as does the level and extent of the lesion and the severity of the neurological deficits. Patients obtain a useful recovery <50% of the time when surgery is delayed for more than 36 h after symptom onset [75]. In one review, only 15/27 recovered completely when surgery was delayed for more than 36 h after symptoms onset [76].

Pearls for Improving Patient Outcomes

- Consider CAD in patients complaining of sudden onset of significant neck pain with history of trauma, however minor. Neurological symptoms may be absent at presentation.
- Assess for a cardiac cause of neck pain, especially in women, and evaluate for other symptoms or risk factors which may suggest coronary artery disease.
- Suspect CEA in patients with significant neck pain and risk factors such as injection drug use, diabetes, immunocompromised, chronic renal failure, cancer, alcoholism, recent distant or contiguous infections, or recent invasive spinal procedure.
- Never rule out meningitis using Kernig's and Brudzinski's signs, as they are poorly sensitive.
- Do not rely on the absence of fever or a normal WBC count alone to rule out infection.
- Do not rule out meningitis using a corrected CSF value for traumatic lumbar punctures.
- Do not rely on plain films to exclude deep neck infections.
- Give immediate antibiotics for suspected meningitis, as delay in antibiotic administration for CT or lumbar puncture significantly increases mortality.
- Arrange specific follow-up for patients with undifferentiated neck masses.
- Exercise caution in incision and drainage of cervical masses in the emergency department due to the possibility of malignancy. Consultation may be advisable.
- Suspect cervical epidural hematoma in a patient with neck pain and radicular symptoms who has any of the following risk factors: anticoagulation, pregnancy, liver disease, rheumatologic disorders, preceding minor trauma or chiropractic manipulation.

References

1. Lee WW, Jensen ER. Bilateral internal carotid artery dissection due to trivial trauma. *J Emerg Med* 2000; 19(1):35–41.

2. Saeed AB, Shuaib A, Al-Sulaiti G, Emery D. Vertebral artery dissection: warning symptoms, clinical features and prognosis in 26 patients. *Can J Neurol Sci* 2000; 27(4):292–6.

3. Dziewas R, Konrad C, Drager B, Evers S, Besselmann M, Ludemann P, Kuhlenbaumer G, Stogbauer F, Ringelstein EB. Cervical artery dissection – clinical features, risk factors, therapy and outcome in 126 patients. *J Neurol* 2003; 250(10):1179–84.

4. Wessels T, Rottger C, Kaps M, Traupe H, Stolz E. Upper cranial nerve palsy resulting from spontaneous carotid dissection. *J Neurol* 2005; 252(4):453–6.

5. Chiche L, Praquin B, Koskas F, Kieffer E. Spontaneous dissection of the extracranial vertebral artery: indications and long-term outcome of surgical treatment. *Ann Vasc Surg* 2005; 19(1):5–10.

6. Wessels T, Sparing R, Neuschaefer-Rube C, Klotzsch C. Vocal cord palsy resulting from spontaneous carotid dissection. *Laryngoscope* 2003; 113(3):537–40.

7. Guidetti D, Pisanello A, Giovanardi F, Morandi C, Zuccoli G, Troiso A. Spontaneous carotid dissection presenting lower cranial nerve palsies. *J Neurol Sci* 2001; 184(2):203–7.

8. Rees JH, Valentine AR, Llewelyn JG. Spontaneous bilateral carotid and vertebral artery dissection presenting as a Collet-Sicard syndrome. *Br J Radiol* 1997; 70(836):856–8.

9. Silbert PL, Mokri B, Schievink WI. Headache and neck pain in spontaneous internal carotid and vertebral artery dissections. *Neurology* 1995; 45(8):1517–22.

10. Mokri B, Houser OW, Sandok BA, Piepgras DG. Spontaneous dissections of the vertebral arteries. *Neurology* 1988; 38(6):880–5.

11. Munera F, Cohn S, Rivas LA. Penetrating injuries of the neck: use of helical computed tomographic angiography. *J Trauma* 2005; 58(2):413–18.

12. Lipetz JS, Ledon J, Silber J. Severe coronary artery disease presenting with a chief complaint of cervical pain. *Am J Phys Med Rehabil* 2003; 82(9):716–20.

13. Chen W, Woods SL, Puntillo KA. Gender differences in symptoms associated with acute myocardial infarction: a review of the research. *Heart Lung* 2005; 34(4):240–7.

14. Cardenas-Malta KR, Cortes-Flores AO, Fuentes-Orozco C, Del Carmen Martinez-Oropeza L, Lopez-Ramirez MK, Gonzalez-Ojeda A. Necrotizing mediastinitis in deep neck infections. *Cir Cir* 2005; 73(4):263–7. [Article in Spanish]

15. McVernon J, Trotter CL, Slack MP, Ramsay ME. Trends in *Haemophilus influenzae* type b infections in adults in England and Wales: surveillance study. *Br Med J* 2004; 329(7467):655–8.

16. Berger G, Landau T, Berger S, Finkelstein Y, Bernheim J, Ophir D. The rising incidence of adult acute epiglottitis and epiglottic abscess. *Am J Otolaryngol* 2003; 24(6):374–83.

17. Wood N, Menzies R, McIntyre P. Epiglottitis in Sydney before and after the introduction of vaccination against *Haemophilus influenzae* type b disease. *Inter Med J* 2005; 35(9):530–5.

18. Shah RK, Roberson DW, Jones DT. Epiglottitis in the *Hemophilus influenzae* type B vaccine era: changing trends. *Laryngoscope* 2004; 114(3):557–60.

19. Williams MF, Eisele DW, Wyatt SH. Neck needle foreign bodies in intravenous drug abusers. *Laryngoscope* 1993; 103(1 Pt 1):59–63.

20. Myers EM, Kirkland LS Jr, Mickey R. The head and neck sequelae of cervical intravenous drug abuse. *Laryngoscope* 1988; 98(2):213–18.

21. Smith MA, Trowers NR, Klein RS. Cervical osteomyelitis caused by Pseudomonas cepacia in an intravenous-drug abuser. *J Clin Microbiol* 1985; 21(3):445–6.

22. Sapico FL, Montgomerie JZ. Vertebral osteomyelitis in intravenous drug abusers: report of three cases and review of the literature. *Rev Infect Dis* 1980; 2(2):196–206.

23. Darouiche RO, Hamill RJ, Greenberg SB, Weathers SW, Musher DM. Bacterial spinal epidural abscess. Review of 43 cases and literature survey. *Medicine (Baltimore)* 1992; 71(6):369–85.

24. Ravicovitch MA, Spallone A. Spinal epidural abscesses: surgical and parasurgical management. *Eur Neurol* 1982; 21:347–57.

25. Durand ML, Calderwood SB, Weber DJ, Miller SI, Southwick FS, Caviness Jr. VS, Swartz MN. Acute bacterial meningitis in adults. A review of 493 episodes.

26. Thomas KE, Hasbun R, Jekel J, Quagliarello VJ. The diagnostic accuracy of Kernig's sign, Brudzinski's sign, and nuchal rigidity in adults with suspected meningitis. *Clin Infect Dis* 2002; 35(1):46–52. Epub 2002 Jun 5.

27. Crespo AN, Chone CT, Fonseca AS, Montenegro MC, Pereira R, Milani JA. Clinical versus computed tomography evaluation in the diagnosis and management of deep neck infection. *Sao Paulo Med J* 2004; 122(6):259–63. Epub 2005 Feb 2.

28. Shah RK, Roberson DW, Jones DT. Epiglottitis in the *Hemophilus influenzae* type B vaccine era: changing trends. *Laryngoscope* 2004; 114(3):557–60.

29. Chang YL, Lo SH, Wang PC, Shu YH. Adult acute epiglottitis: experiences in a Taiwanese setting. *Otolaryngol Head Neck Surg* 2005; 132(5):689–93.

30. Proulx N, Frechette D, Toye B, Chan J, Kravcik S. Delays in the administration of antibiotics are associated with mortality from adult acute bacterial meningitis. *Q J Med* 2005; 98(4):291–8. Epub 2005 Mar 10.

31. van de Beek D, de Gans J, Spanjaard L, Weisfelt M, Reitsma JB, Vermeulen M. Clinical features and prognostic factors in adults with bacterial meningitis. *N Engl J Med* 2004; 351(18):1849–59.

32. Rigamonti D, Liem L, Sampath P, Knoller N, Namaguchi Y, Schreibman DL, Sloan MA, Wolf A, Zeidman S. Spinal epidural abscess: contemporary trends in etiology, evaluation, and management. *Surg Neurol* 1999; 52(2):189–96.

33. Redekop GJ, Del Maestro RF. Diagnosis and management of spinal epidural abscess. *Can J Neurol Sci* 1992; 19(2):180–7.

34. Ekbom DC, D-Elia J, Isaacson B, Lamarca F, Chepeha DB, Bradford CR. Spinal epidural abscess after cervical pharyngoesophageal dilation. *Head Neck* 2005; 27(6):543–8.

35. Jerrard DA, Olshaker J. Simultaneous uvulitis and epiglottitis without fever or leukocytosis. *Am J Emerg Med* 1996; 14(6):551–2.

36. Bonsu BK, Harper MB. A low peripheral blood white blood cell count in infants younger than 90 days increases the odds of acute bacterial meningitis relative to bacteremia. *Acad Emerg Med* 2004; 11(12):1297–301.

37. Aronin SI, Peduzzi P, Quagliarello VJ. Community-acquired bacterial meningitis: risk stratification for adverse clinical outcome and effect of antibiotic timing. *Ann Intern Med* 1998; 129(11):862–9.

38. Wong D, Raymond NJ. Spinal epidural abscess. *NZ Med J* 1998; 111:345–7.

39. Bonsu BK, Harper MB. Accuracy and test characteristics of ancillary tests of cerebrospinal fluid for predicting acute bacterial meningitis in children with low white blood cell counts in cerebrospinal fluid. *Acad Emerg Med* 2005; 12(4):303–9.

40. Bonsu BK, Harper MB. Differentiating acute bacterial meningitis from acute viral meningitis among children with cerebrospinal fluid pleocytosis: a multivariable regression model. *Pediatr Infect Dis J* 2004; 23(6):511–7.

41. Nigrovic LE, Kuppermann N, Malley R. Development and validation of a multivariable predictive model to distinguish bacterial from aseptic meningitis in children in the post-*Haemophilus influenzae* era. *Pediatrics* 2002; 110(4):712–19.

42. Freedman SB, Marrocco A, Pirie J, Dick PT. Predictors of bacterial meningitis in the era after *Haemophilus influenzae*. *Arch Pediatr Adolesc Med* 2001; 155(12):1301–6.

43. Mayefsky JH, Roghmann KJ. Determination of leukocytosis in traumatic spinal tap specimens. *Am J Med* 1987; 82(6):1175–81.

44. Nemzek WR, Katzberg RW, Van Slyke MA, Bickley LS. A reappraisal of the radiologic findings of acute inflammation of the epiglottis and supraglottic structures in adults. *Am J Neuroradiol* 1995; 16(3):495–502.

45. Smith MM, Mukherji SK, Thompson JE, Castillo M. CT in adult supraglottitis. *Am J Neuroradiol* 1996; 17(7):1355–8.

46. Boucher C, Dorion D, Fisch C. Retropharyngeal abscesses: a clinical and radiologic correlation. *J Otolaryngol* 1999; 28(3):134–7.

47. Nagy M, Backstrom J. Comparison of the sensitivity of lateral neck radiographs and computed tomography scanning in pediatric deep-neck infections. *Laryngoscope* 1999; 109(5):775–9.

48. Palme CE, Lowinger D, Petersen AJ. Fish bones at the cricopharyngeus: a comparison of plain-film radiology and computed tomography. *Laryngoscope* 1999; 109(12):1955–8.

49. Lue AJ, Fang WD, Manolidis S. Use of plain radiography and computed tomography to identify fish bone foreign bodies. *Otolaryngol Head Neck Surg* 2000; 123(4):435–8.

50. Vural C, Gungor A, Comerci S. Accuracy of computerized tomography in deep neck infections in the pediatric population. *Am J Otolaryngol* 2003; 24(3):143–8.

51. Stone ME, Walner DL, Koch BL, Egelhoff JC, Myer CM. Correlation between computed tomography and surgical findings in retropharyngeal inflammatory processes in children. *Int J Pediatr Otorhinolaryngol* 1999; 49(2):121–5.

52. Curry WT, Hoh BL, Amin-Hanjani S, Eskandar EN. Spinal epidural abscess: clinical presentation, management, and outcome. *Surg Neurol* 2005; 63(4):364–71.

53. Williams JW, Powell T. Epidural abscess of the cervical spine: case report and literature review. *Br J Radiol* 1990; 63(751):576–8.

54. Gourin CG, Johnson JT. Incidence of unsuspected metastases in lateral cervical cysts. *Laryngoscope* 2000; 110(10 Pt 1):1637–41.

55. Bhattacharyya N. Predictive factors for neoplasia and malignancy in a neck mass. *Arch Otolaryngol Head Neck Surg* 1999; 125(3):303–7.

56. Eskey CJ, Robson CD, Weber AL. Imaging of benign and malignant soft tissue tumors of the neck. *Radiol Clin N Am* 2000; 38(5):1091–104.

57. Josephson GD, Spencer WR, Josephson JS. Thyroglossal duct cyst: the New York Eye and Ear Infirmary experience and a literature review. *Ear Nose Throat J* 1998; 77(8):642–4, 646–7, 651.

58. Gritzmann N, Hollerweger A, Macheiner P, Rettenbacher T. Sonography of soft tissue masses of the neck. *J Clin Ultrasound* 2001; 30(6):356–73.

59. Mighell AJ, High AS. Histological identification of carcinoma in 21 gauge needle tracks after fine needle aspiration biopsy of head and neck carcinoma. *J Clin Pathol* 1998; 51(3):241–3.

60. Lydiatt DD. Medical malpractice and cancer of the larynx. *Laryngoscope* 2002; 112(3):445–8.

61. Demierre B, Unger PF, Bongioanni F. Sudden cervical pain: spontaneous cervical epidural hematoma. *Am J Emerg Med* 1991; 9(1):54–6.

62. Williams JM, Allegra JR. Spontaneous cervical epidural hematoma. *Ann Emerg Med* 1994; 23(6):1368–70.

63. Stoll A, Sanchez M. Epidural hematoma after epidural block: implications for its use in pain management. *Surg Neurol* 2002; 57(4):235–40.

64. Tender GC, Awasthi D. Spontaneous cervical spinal epidural hematoma in a 12-year old girl: case report and review of the literature. *J La State Med Soc* 2004; 156(4):196–8.

65. Steinmetz MP, Kalfas IH, Willis B, Chalavi A, Harlan RC. Successful surgical management of a case of spontaneous epidural hematoma of the spine during pregnancy. *Spine J* 2003; 3(6):539–42.

66. Ferry P, Reisner C, Ashpole R. A case of spontaneous cervical extradural haematoma. *Hosp Med* 2001; 62(7):436–7.

67. Vaya A, Resureccion M, Ricart JM, Ortuno C, Ripoll F, Mira Y, Aznar J. *Clin Appl Thromb Hemost* 2001; 7(2):166–8.

68. Lobitz B, Grate I. Acute epidural hematoma of the cervical spine: an unusual cause of neck pain. *South Med J* 1995; 88(5):580–2.

69. Nagel MA, Taff IP, Cantos EL, Patel MP, Maytal J, Berman D. Spontaneous spinal epidural hematoma in a 7-year-old girl. Diagnostic value of magnetic resonance imaging. *Clin Neurol Neurosurg* 1989; 91(2):157–60.

70. Lin IY. Diagnostic pitfall: nontraumatic spinal epidural hematoma mimicking a brainstem stroke. *Ann Emerg Med* 2004; 44(2):183–4.

71. Saxler G, Barden B. Extensive spinal epidural hematoma—an uncommon entity following cervical chiropractic manipulation. *Z Orthop Ihre Grenzgeb* 2004; 142(1):79–82.

72. Segal DH, Lidov MW, Camins MB. Cervical epidural hematoma after chiropractic manipulation in a healthy young woman: case report. *Neurosurgery* 1996; 39(5):1043–5.

73. Zupruk GM, Mehta Z. Brown-sequard syndrome associated with posttraumatic cervical epidural hematoma: case report and review of the literature. *Neurosurgery* 1989; 25(2):278–80.

74. Sakamoto N, Yanaka K, Matsumaru Y, Nose T. Cervical epidural hematoma causing hemiparesis. *Arch Neurol* 2003; 60(5):783.

75. McDonnell GV, Bell KE, Hawkins SA. A pain in the neck. *Postgrad Med J* 2000; 76(891):229–30.

76. Patel H, Boaz JC, Phillips JP, Garg BP. Spontaneous spinal epidural hematoma in children. *Pediatr Neurol* 1998; 19(4):302–7.

Chapter 7 | **Trauma Management in the ED**

David E. Manthey & Bret A. Nicks

Introduction

Emergency medicine physicians (EPs) provide the initial trauma care of most trauma patients. Although we often work in concert with the trauma surgeons on the more seriously injured patients, it behooves us to be on the cutting edge of trauma care for all of our injured patients. Several pitfalls that frequently surface as areas of concern for many EPs are addressed here.

Pitfall | **Failure to implement surrogates to crystalloid during resuscitation**

Crystalloid fluid resuscitation is crucial to maintain perfusion to vital organs. It is important, however, to frequently reassess the patient between boluses to determine whether he/she is a responder, partial responder, or non-responder to the fluids. This allows one to determine the need for blood products, surgical intervention, or other therapies. Therefore, infusing predetermined boluses of fluid is essential to allowing one to determine whether alternate therapies need be initiated.

Overzealous fluid administration can have several deleterious physiologic effects. Elevating the blood pressure above the tamponade pressure of post-traumatic clot formation may cause clot disruption and worsen bleeding and thus shock. Also, hemodilution causing a progressive anemia decreases the oxygen carrying capacity of the intravascular space and decreases the viscosity of the blood allowing it to more easily elute around an incomplete thrombus [1]. By judiciously utilizing fluid resuscitation, selecting and implementing proper blood products or surrogates when required (red blood cells (RBC), plasma, platelets, clotting factors, rFVIIa), and better monitoring the response to fluids, we should be able to improve outcomes by limiting further hemorrhage and minimizing the complications of hemodilution.

> KEY FACT | **Patients must be reassessed regularly after boluses of predefined quantities of crystalloid. Only by doing so can the need for other adjuncts be identified.**

As optimal perfusion pressure must be maintained, elevation of the blood pressure above that of the tamponade pressure of the clot may be required. In doing so, a clinical trade off is

made and must be recognized. This allows for more aggressive management of the point of active bleeding, as well as resuscitation with oxygen carrying products to replace the lost hemoglobin. Administration of other perfusion adjuncts can minimize the volume of crystalloid necessary to maintain perfusion. The rapidity of which definitive hemorrhage control is established is paramount to the survival of the patient. Likewise, identifying and controlling a bleeding source is critical to minimize ongoing blood loss.

Pitfall | **Over-reliance on focused abdominal sonography in trauma**

Focused abdominal sonography in trauma (FAST) examinations has rapidly replaced diagnostic peritoneal lavage (DPL) in the evaluation of unstable or stable trauma patients as part of the primary or secondary survey. Multiple studies have reported the sensitivity of the FAST examination for determining the presence of intra-abdominal fluid to be 90%, with a specificity of 99%, and an accuracy of 98% [2–4]. As such, the FAST examination has its primary utility in the unstable trauma patient who should not go to computed tomography (CT) scan, but rather the operating room due to increased suspicion for intra-abdominal injury as the cause of instability. In patients who are hypotensive after blunt abdominal trauma and not hemodynamically stable enough to undergo diagnostic CT, negative US findings virtually exclude intra-abdominal surgical injury as the cause of hemodynamic instability, while positive US findings indicate surgical injury in approximately 70% of cases [5]. The FAST examination also may be helpful in a multi-patient trauma to triage critically ill patients when not all can get a CT scan in a timely manner.

> KEY FACT | **In stable patients, a negative FAST examination does not obviate the need for CT and a positive one does not mandate operative intervention.**

In general, a positive FAST examination in the stable patient does not mandate surgical intervention as non-operative management for a solid organ injury may be indicated based on patient stability, age, physiologic reserve, and severity of injury based on CT grading. When indicated, CT imaging of the stable patient is obtained regardless of the FAST examination. A single negative FAST examination must be regarded as only one snapshot of a patient's condition at the time it was taken. There may be limited fluid from a bowel injury in the initial period, a contained sub-capsular hemorrhage that would not result in identifiable free fluid, or a delayed rupture of a solid organ only identified on subsequent examinations.

FAST examinations are less invasive but as a sensitive test as DPL for hemoperitoneum and as such should replace the DPL in the evaluation of a trauma patient. They should not however, take the place of repeat physical examinations or a CT scan.

Pitfall | Not recognizing the significance of a "seat-belt sign" and over-reliance on the CT scan

> KEY FACT | Patients with lower abdominal bruising from seat-belt impact are at high risk for serious injuries that are often not identified on abdominal CT.

Patients with blunt abdominal trauma who have a "seat-belt sign" have an increased incidence of abdominal injury [6–8]. The "seat-belt syndrome" denotes a pattern of injuries in the plane of the lap belt. The injuries to the spine, vasculature, and solid organs can be identified on CT. However, the list of injuries includes small and large bowel injuries for which CT is only up to 74% sensitive in children, especially early in the evaluation [7]. This is an important point to remember even without a seat-belt sign. Extravasation of contrast is rarely seen in a patient with perforated bowel due to blunt trauma. In one study, 21% of adult patients with a seat-belt sign had a small bowel perforation, while only 1.9% had it without a seat-belt sign [8]. This would suggest that repeated clinical examinations and observation would be indicated for these patients. Without good data about the adverse effects of waiting or the current sensitivity and specificity of DPL for bowel injury, it is presently hard to define a better approach.

Pitfall | Failure to recognize early shock in the geriatric trauma patient

Geriatric patients have several reasons that diminish the normal response of tachycardia to hypovolemia. The physiologic reserve or ability of the elderly heart due to age or prior myocardial pathology may limit its response. Polypharmacy, most notably the use of beta blockers, calcium channel blockers, and other negative chronotropic drugs may prevent responsive tachycardia. These physiologic limitations may create a false sense of assurance because of "normal" vital signs in a patient that would otherwise be tachycardic. Good

clinical acumen and elevated suspicion are warranted as these patients require an efficient, focused work-up, stabilization, and disposition to an appropriate intermediate or intensive care unit (ICU) level of care [1].

Pitfall | Withholding radiographic studies in the pregnant trauma patient for fear of fetal radiation exposure

> KEY FACT | Pregnant patients should not have indicated radiographic studies withheld. Used judiciously, the radiation dose is not significant. Optimizing the mother's treatment will affect the best outcomes for both patients.

Fear over fetal radiation exposure has led to withholding indicated radiographic studies in pregnant patients. An educated decision on the use of imaging in the pregnant trauma patient should supplant any protocol or fear of use and be made in context with current knowledge about radiation exposure and the risk to the fetus. The National Council on Radiation Protection Report No. 54 states: "The risk (of abnormality) is considered to be negligible at 5 rad (50 mGy) or less when compared to other risks of pregnancy, and the risk of malformations is substantially increased above controls only at doses above 15 rad (150 mGy)." The American College of Obstetricians and Gynecologists states "... exposure to less than 5000 mrad (50 mGy) has not been associated with an increase in fetal anomalies or pregnancy loss." This is a cumulative dose over the duration of pregnancy. The fetus is most sensitive to malformations and teratogenesis at 2–15 weeks after conception. The radiation exposure to the fetus by various studies is listed below [9, 10].

Radiograph		CT	
Imaging	mGy	Imaging	mGy
C-spine	<0.1	Head	0.05
Chest	<0.0001	Chest	0.16
Pelvis	2	Abdomen	8
Lumbar spine	4	Pelvis	25
Hip and femur	3	Lumbar spine	35

The physician should always consider if use of a modality with less radiation exposure (ultrasound) will yield the same information. Always assess the risk-to-benefit ratio for the patient and the fetus. The patient should be informed of the risk, albeit minimal, of the radiographic studies. Use of radiographic studies should be based on the stability of the patient, degree of suspicion, and risk of injury.

Pitfall | **Inappropriate use of CTs and plain radiographs of the spine**

> **KEY FACT | With newer CT scanners, spinal CTs can be reformatted from abdominal CTs. Because of its superior sensitivity, patients in whom there is high suspicion for spinal injury should have spinal CT.**

Less than 50% of current academic emergency departments continue to obtain additional lumbar and thoracic spine plain films after obtaining a CT of the chest and abdomen. These additional radiographs occur at additional expense and radiation to the patient without additional diagnostic value. The CT images can be reformatted to deliver images of the spinal column with a sensitivity of 97% for thoracic spine fractures and 95% for lumbar spine fractures. The CT may miss nonoperative compression fractures. The sensitivity of plain radiographs is 62% for the thoracic spine and 86% for the lumbar spine [11]. Two recent reviews of more than 3000 patients suggest that plain radiographs of the spine should no longer be utilized in the trauma patient as CT has supplanted that radiographic modality [12]. The charges and dose of radiation must be taken into consideration with plain films charge about $145, and delivering 6.36 mSv of radiation and CT charge about $880 and delivering 19.42 mSv CT for imaging of the lumbar spine [13]. Due to the additional radiation exposure and cost for CT, perhaps a more rational approach may be to reserve CT for those in whom it is not possible to obtain adequate plain films or those with a high suspicion of injury, however, further research will be required to best identify a risk stratifying approach.

Pitfall | **Failure to appropriately apply C-spine clearance rules**

Two C-spine clearance rules have come to the forefront in recent years, the NEXUS rule and the Canadian C-spine rule. Without getting into the discussion of which might be better, the authors would like to emphasize the limitations of such rules in general. We can all recall that NEXUS requires a patient to have normal level of alertness, but how many can define what that really means. The NEXUS study defines it as an altered level of alertness which can include any of the following:

1. Glasgow Coma Scale (GCS) score of 14 or less.
2. Disorientation to person, place, time, or events.
3. Inability to remember three objects at 5 min.
4. Delayed or inappropriate response to external stimuli.

This is not a downfall of the study, it is an issue with how we often oversimplify a rule to make it easier to apply and therefore utilize. But the NEXUS authors looked at their criteria and state it best: "Because each of the five low-risk criteria was the only marker of non-low-risk status in at least a few patients with significant cervical spine injury, modification of the overall NEXUS decision instrument by eliminating any one of the criteria would markedly reduce sensitivity and make the instrument unacceptable for clinical use [14]."

Neither rule unambiguously defines distracting injuries. A recent study suggests that proximity of injury due to the gating theory that a noxious stimuli from the upper extremity may provide enough counter-irritation through the spinal pain pathways that other pain signals may go unnoticed [15]. This may make upper extremity injuries distracting even if they don't fit the guidelines of either NEXUS or the Canadian C-spine rules.

The Canadian C-spine rule removes anyone over the age of 64. The NEXUS rule does not, and has looked at the geriatric population of the study citing a sensitivity of the NEXUS criteria for all cervical spine injuries in the geriatric group of 98.5% (95% CI, 94.8–99.7%), and the sensitivity for clinically significant injury was 100% (95% CI, 97.1–100%). There are various case reports of elderly patients with injury, but they often cite inappropriate evaluation of the level of alertness. The NEXUS group urged caution in using the criteria among children, especially those younger than 9 as there was a limited number of patients and injuries in this group. The Canadian C-spine rule was for patients 16 years and older.

The Canadian C-spine rule [16] included the presence of a concerning mechanism (fall from 1 m or greater, axial load to head, motorized recreational vehicles, bicycle collision, or motor vehicle collision (MVC) with high speed, rollover, or ejection). The NEXUS study recognized that it was not utilizing a criterion for mechanism but all of these were certainly included in the group that was studied.

The goal of both of these rules is to decrease the use of unnecessary radiographs in the evaluation of the cervical spine in blunt trauma. We doubt that either group wanted their algorithms to supplant good clinical acumen and judgment. Nevertheless, appropriate application of these rules can identify patients at risk for cervical spine injury while significantly reducing the number of cervical spine X-rays necessary and should be encouraged. When doing so, however, it is imperative that the clinician know how to apply the rules appropriately.

Pitfall | **Failure to obtain CT imaging of the cervical spine in patients at high risk for injury**

> **KEY FACT | Because of its superior sensitivity, patients in whom there is high suspicion for spinal injury should have spinal CT.**

The three-view cervical series has anatomical and technical limitations, particularly at the craniocervical and cervicothoracic junctions, making 25–50% of films inadequate. This is particularly evident in the unconscious polytrauma victims where image quality decreases secondary to tracheal tube or collar artifact. Adequate plain radiographs have a sensitivity of only 52%, a specificity of 98%, a positive predictive value of 81%, and a negative predictive value of 93%. Helical CT had a sensitivity and specificity of 98%, a positive predictive value of 89%, and a negative predictive value of >99% [17]. In patients with altered mental status, polytrauma, or in which there is a high index of suspicion for potential injury, CT scanning will provide better imaging than plain radiographs [18, 19].

The argument over additional costs of CT versus radiograph has been looked at based on institutional cost (insurance, legal action due to missed fractures and disability, etc.) with CT being cost-effective even if plain radiographs were 90% sensitive. In one study, the need for supplemental CT imaging of the cervical spine in up to 62% of trauma patients due to the inadequacy of plain radiographs [18]. Based on this data, especially in urban trauma centers, CT scan of the neck should be the imaging modality of choice in the aforementioned situations when imaging is needed. However, in patients with neurologic deficits and a negative CT scan, further evaluation often necessitates an MRI.

Pitfall | Failure to screen for blunt carotid injury in patients at risk

Data previously supported screening asymptomatic trauma patients for blunt cerebrovascular injury (BCVI) to prevent associated neurologic sequelae [20, 21]. Aggressive angiographic screening for BCVI based on a patient's injury pattern and symptoms allows for early diagnosis and treatment and is cost-effective because it prevents ischemic neurological events (INEs). Angiography, however is time-consuming and necessitates transfer of a potentially unstable patient to an angiographic suite. Duplex Doppler US has many features of a promising screening tool for BCVI: rapidity, mobility, cost-effectiveness, and non-invasiveness. Like focused abdominal sonography for trauma, it can be performed simultaneously in resuscitation, clearing of other torso injuries, and temporary fixation of fractures. However, several studies have shown US has inadequate sensitivity to help rule out this condition when compared with CT angiography [22]. The notable morbidity with missed dissections warrants routine contrast-enhanced studies of the carotid and vertebral vessels when injury is suspected in blunt trauma patients with direct injury to the neck, evidence of ecchymosis or swelling over vascular structures, or neurologic deficits not otherwise explained.

Pitfall | Reliance on a dopplerable pulse to rule out vascular injury

Current literature supports that there can be adequate flow for a Doppler signal despite having an important arterial injury proximally during the evaluation for occult arterial injury from penetrating proximal extremity trauma. Doppler pressure indices (Ankle–Brachial Index (ABI) or Brachial–Brachial Index (BBI)) have a sensitivity of 72.5%, a specificity of 100%, a positive predictive value of 100%, and a negative predictive value of 96%. Depending on the level of concern, advancing to duplex sonography or arteriography may be indicated. Careful and repeated clinical examination and ABI/BBI indices are pivotal for early diagnosis of present or developing injury [23, 24]. Early diagnosis and timely treatment of extremity vascular injuries are essential if limb salvage and limb function are to be optimized.

Pitfall | Failure to intervene selectively on incidentally identified pneumothoraces

> KEY FACT | As previously undetected pneumothoraces are being identified on CT scans, clinicians must identify those that would benefit from intervention.

The number of patients undergoing abdominal CT during their trauma evaluation is increasing. CT is more accurate than plain radiographs in the detection of pneumothoracies [25]. With the increased sensitivity, it is not uncommon to identify incidental small pneumothoraces that would otherwise have been undetected with plain radiography. CT-directed size classification allows grading of occult pneumothoraces. Miniscule refers to air collections less than 1cm thick and on less than five contiguous 10-mm slices. Anterior pneumothoraces are defined as air collections . 1cm thick, on five or more contiguous 10-mm slices, and not extending to the mid-coronal line. Anterolateral pneumothoraces extended to the mid-coronal line or beyond and therefore are larger than the defined anterior pneumothorax. [26].

Classification of pneumothoraces by size

Miniscule	Air collections less than 1 cm thick and that appear on less than five contiguous 10 mm slices
Anterior	Air collections >1 cm thick and that appear on five or more contiguous slices but do not extend to the mid-coronal line
Anterolateral	Extend to the mid-coronal line or beyond and are therefore larger than anterior pneumothoraces

Because many of these small pneumothoraces would likely have resorbed spontaneously and are therefore clinically insignificant, it is important to selectively intervene only on those that are likely to benefit. The stability of the patient, the degree of patient's symptoms, the current size of the pneumothorax, the change in size over time, the etiology of the pneumothorax, and the degree of underlying lung disease must all be considered when deciding whether to intervene.

Treatment with tube thoracostomy should be considered in occult pneumothoraces found in trauma patients if they are more than anterior in size, the patient is undergoing positive pressure ventilation, those associated with underlying lung disease, or if the patient is considered unstable. A stable patient has been described as one with a respiratory rate of <24 bpm, a heart rate between 60 and 120 bpm, a normal blood pressure, room air saturations greater than 90%, and can speak in full sentences between breaths [27].

Pitfall | **Avoiding succinylcholine in the acutely burned or crushed patient**

> KEY FACT | **Patients with significant burns are not at risk for succinylcholine-induced hyperkalemia until 5 days after the injury.**

The concern in a burn or crush victim is the pathologic hyperkalemic response associated succinylcholine. However, this response is caused by receptor up-regulation which takes about 5 days post injury to occur but lasts an indefinable period of time. As well, there has been no correlation between the percent of body surface area burned and the likelihood of this hyperkalemic response, especially in acute injuries. As most intubations in the ED occur well within the 5-day window, it is safe and more appropriate to utilize succinylcholine due to its rapidity of onset and short duration of action unmatched by any non-depolarizing agent. If, for some reason, the patient arrives needing to be intubated after several days, a non-depolarizing agent such as rocuronium or vecuronium would be advised. Recall that the up-regulated immature nicotinic receptors are relatively refractory to non-depolarizing agents and therefore may require larger doses for appropriate rapid sequence intubation (RSI) response.

Pitfall | **Failure to provide pelvic compression for open book pelvic fractures**

> KEY FACT | **Unstable patients with pelvic fractures should have a pelvic compression device placed if their bleeding source is not in their abdomen.**

Circumferential pelvic compression is a standard component of the acute stabilization of patients with pelvic fractures. This is initiated in the pre-hospital setting, as well as in the

ED until stabilization and definitive management can be established. Recent compression devices have been introduced that provide consistent compression force better pelvic closure and stabilization than standard sheet technique and at least one can be set to specific amount of torque. By decreasing the intra-pelvic volume the potential blood loss is reduced, minimizing subsequent hypovolemic shock [28]. Application of these simple corset devices is easy and rapid, and does not interfere with subsequent radiographic imaging. The device will aid in controlling venous bleeding. However, if the patient remains unstable, an arteriogram to evaluate for and treat arterial bleeding may be indicated.

Pitfall | **Discharging a mild head injury patient with a normal head CT and GCS score of 15 without close observation**

The term "mild head injury" is used to denote amnesia or a loss of consciousness from a closed head injury. Current management protocols for mild head injury include observation, helical CT, or frequently a combination of both [29]. Several studies addressing patients presenting to the emergency department that have regained a normal level of consciousness, have no abnormal neurologic findings, lack additional body system injuries, and have a normal acute helical head CT state that home management is appropriate [30, 31]. The key to this approach is continued and appropriate observation of the patient. Variables not completely addressed in these studies were CT misinterpretations, and social factors limiting the level of outpatient home care. Further consideration of available home monitoring, distance from the nearest care facility, and those on concurrent anticoagulation is crucial prior to discharge.

Important Issues That Lack Formal Data

Pitfall | **Inappropriate choice of vascular access**

Vascular access can be accomplished via two large bore peripheral intravenous (i.v.) lines. The rate of flow through a 14 g antecubital is twice that of a 16 g central venous catheter due to pressure and the catheter length. In the absence of peripheral lines, the placement of an 8.5 French sheath introducer centrally will allow for faster administration of resuscitative fluids and blood products than a triple lumen. As for the location of the line, there is significant debate. The femoral access is logistically easiest because it is remote from any airway and thoracic evaluation and resuscitative efforts (intubation, chest tubes, etc.) as well as unhindered by the cervical collar. However, it carries a significantly higher rate of venous thrombosis and infection when compared to a subclavian line. Subclavian line thrombosis rate are between 1.5% and

12.5% whereas femoral line thrombosis rates reach up to 25% [32]. Catheter-related clinical sepsis is only 1.5% in subclavian catheters, while it approaches 4.4% in femoral catheters [33]. In the clinical situation of hemodynamic instability with inability to obtain peripheral access, the femoral line should be utilized, but promptly replaced when the clinical situation improves.

Pitfall | Failure to remove patients from backboards

> KEY FACT | Patients should be removed from backboards as soon as possible.

Formal data gives us three significant points of information. First is that the backboard does not adequately stabilize the spine, nor maintain it in the appropriate position any better than lying flat on the gurney. Log rolling minimizes excessive movement of the patient's spine. Finally, even in healthy patients, increased duration of time on a backboard leads to increased discomfort and poor tissue oxygenation [34]. Backboards allow the convenient transport of a patient from the emergency medical services (EMS) stretcher to the gurney without detriment to the spine. Removal from the backboard rapidly after transfer, CT, or radiographic imaging improves patient comfort without detriment to spine care, and possibly decreases skin breakdown [35, 36].

Pitfall | Errors in transporting patients to tertiary care facilities

The answer to this depends on the degree of certainty that an injury has occurred, and the transferring facilities ability to both diagnose and initiate treatment of the injury. Transporting all trauma patients to regional trauma centers is inefficient; however, the bypass of nearer, non-designated hospitals in deference to regional trauma centers decreases mortality in the severely injured [37–39]. In general, after the initial assessment, the transferring facility should initiate the transfer as soon as possible. Appropriate stabilization of the ABC's of a trauma patient should always be undertaken and therefore at least a CXR should be done to evaluate for a pneumothorax (PTX). Appropriate resuscitation should continue before, during, and after the transfer. Blood products can be sent with the patient if they are available.

Radiographic studies are often repeated at the accepting institution even if they can accompany the patient on CD or via the Internet. Postponing a transfer in order to perform these studies delays the evaluation at the center that can address any life-threatening issues. Continuing the work-up while awaiting the transfer team and transferring all data and images with them can quicken the involvement of the appropriate subspecialty team. Sending the patients without a full radiographic evaluation will increase the number who arrive at tertiary care centers but do not require specialty intervention, but that is the necessary and acceptable cost of an aggressive stance in the treatment of trauma.

Pitfall | Over-Reliance on laboratory data in trauma

In most cases of trauma, laboratory data has minimal utility. A complete blood count can be misleading, as it only tells you the state of the intravascular concentration of RBC at the time of the draw. Therefore it tells you the state of anemia, but not whether or not the patient bled a significant amount, or whether or not there is ongoing hemorrhage. A subsequent CBC to identify any change from the initial CBC is essential. An electrolyte panel is most commonly normal or not relevant to the care of the patient unless a concurrent co-morbid condition caused the traumatic event. Amylase is neither sensitive nor specific in the evaluation of a pancreatic or viscous injury. A type and screen are important if the use of blood products is being considered. However, point-of-care laboratory assessment, and more importantly the trend in the patient's laboratories associated with their clinical course remain most valuable. In the hemodynamically unstable patient, the emphasis should be on resuscitation and blood draws for laboratories should not be allowed to interfere with this.

Pitfall | Intubation of trauma patients with an endotracheal tube (ETT) that is too small

When intubating a trauma patient, keep in mind that the patient may need to undergo instrumentation of the endotracheal tube for cultures or bronchoscopy. Smaller tubes limit the ability of these evaluations, and are more prone to mucopurulent plugging from airway secretions as early as 24 hours post-intubation [40]. Placement of the largest tube possible is beneficial to both future treatment and ventilation weaning of trauma or ICU patients.

Pitfall | Failure to provide adequate analgesia to trauma patients

Under-treatment of pain in the emergency department has received notable attention over the past years. Studies have documented an increase in the use of analgesics, but little evidence supports whether the treatment provides adequate analgesia. The i.v. morphine is considered the criterion standard for the treatment of severe pain. Although morphine given in a single dose of 0.1 mg/kg is the appropriate weight-based dose, fear and overestimation of potential respiratory depression or hypotension lead to suboptimal doses amongst clinicians. The efficacy of 0.1 mg/kg of i.v. morphine to decrease the pain in half approaches only 33% – without any significant adverse effects [41]. Appropriate treatment, not inadequate analgesia, should remain the goal and may require re-education of physicians and nurses.

Pearls for Improving Patient Outcomes

- Patients should be reassessed between crystalloid boluses to determine the best resuscitation strategy.
- FAST examination do not replace CT in stable patients.
- Up to 21% of patients with a seat-belt sign may have hollow viscous injuries, for which CT is only 76% sensitive.
- Elderly patients may not show tachycardia in the face of shock due to medications and underlying physiology.
- Indicated radiographic studies should be obtained on pregnant patients.
- C-spine clearance rules should be used appropriately and in the proper population to obtain the same negative predictive value.
- Doppler pulse alone in a higher-risk patient does not rule out vascular injury in the trauma patient.
- Occult pneumothoraces found on CT may not need intervention.
- Succinylcholine is still paralytic of choice in acutely burned patients.
- Open book pelvic fractures should be treated with a compression device.
- Despite a normal GCS and head CT, mild head injury patients deserve continued monitoring, even in home settings.
- Most trauma patients can be resuscitated with two large bore peripheral i.v. access lines.
- Trauma patients should be removed from backboards as soon as possible for comfort and to prevent skin breakdown.
- Critically ill trauma patients should be transferred to trauma centers after limited life-sustaining interventions without delay for further evaluation.
- Most laboratory data has limited utility in a trauma patient.
- Utilization of a larger size ETT tube facilitates future airway management and evaluation.
- Pain should be treated with adequate analgesia with relevant regard to hemodynamic stability.

References

1. Scalea TM, Simon HM, Duncan AO, et al. Geriatric blunt multiple trauma: improved survival with early invasive monitoring. *J Trauma* 1990; 30(2):129–34; discussion 134–6.
2. Rozycki GS, Ochsner MG, Schmidt JA, et al. A prospective study of surgeon-performed ultrasound as the primary adjunct modality for injured patient assessment. *J Trauma* 1995; 39:492–500.
3. Ma OJ, Mateer JR, Ogata M, et al. Prospective analysis of a rapid trauma ultrasound examination performed by emergency physicians. *J Trauma* 1995; 38:879–85.
4. Hoffman R, Nerlich M, Muggia-Sullam M, et al. Blunt abdominal trauma in cases of multiple trauma evaluated by ultrasonography: a prospective analysis of 291 patients. *J Trauma* 1992; 32:452–8.
5. Farahmand N, Sirlin CB, Brown MA, et al. Hypotensive patients with blunt abdominal trauma: performance of screening US. *Radiology* 235(2):436–43.
6. Sokolove PE, Kuppermann N, Holmes JF. Association between the "seat belt sign" and intra-abdominal injury in children with blunt torso trauma. *Acad Emerg Med* 2005; 12:808–13.
7. Albanese CT, Meza MP, Gardner MJ, et al. Is computed tomography a useful adjunct to the clinical examination for the diagnosis of pediatric gastrointestinal perforation from blunt abdominal trauma in children? *J Trauma* 1996; 40(3):417–21.
8. Wotherspoon S, Chu K, Brown AF. Abdominal injury and the seat-belt sign. *Emerg Med* 2001; 13(1):61–65.
9. Toppenberg KS, Hill DA, Miller DP. Safety of radiographic imaging during pregnancy. *Am Fam Physician* 1999; 59(7):1813–8, 1820.
10. Parry RA, Glaze SA, Archer BR. The AAPM/RSNA physics tutorial for residents. Typical patient radiation doses in diagnostic radiology. *Radiographics* 1999; 19(5):1289–302.
11. Sheridan R, Peralta R, Rhea J, et al. Reformatted visceral protocol helical computed tomographic scanning allows conventional radiographs of the thoracic and lumbar spine to be eliminated in the evaluation of blunt trauma patients. *J Trauma* 2003; 55(4):665–9.
12. Hauser CJ, Visvikis G, Hinrichs C, et al. Prospective validation of computed tomographic screening of the thoracolumbar spine in trauma. *J Trauma* 2003; 55(2):228–34.
13. Wintermark M, Mouhsine E, Theumann N, et al. Thoracolumbar spine fractures in patients who have sustained severe trauma: depiction with multi-detector row CT. *Radiology* 2003; 227(3):681–9.
14. Panacek EA, Mower WR, Holmes JF, et al. NEXUS Group. Test performance of the individual NEXUS low-risk clinical screening criteria for cervical spine injury. *Ann Emerg Med* 2001; 38(1):22–25.
15. Heffernan DS, Schermer CR, Lu SW. What defines a distracting injury in cervical spine assessment? *J Trauma* 2005; 59(6): 1396–9.
16. Bandiera G, Stiell IG, Wells GA, et al. Canadian C-Spine and CT Head Study Group. The Canadian c-spine rule performs better than unstructured physician judgment. *Ann Emerg Med* 2003; 42(3):395–402.
17. McCulloch PT, France J, Jones DL, et al. Helical computed tomography alone compared with plain radiographs with adjunct computed tomography to evaluate the cervical spine after high-energy trauma. *J Bone Joint Surg Am* 2005; 87(11): 2388–94.
18. Gale SC, Gracias PH, Reilly PM, et al. The inefficiency of plain radiography to evaluate the cervical spine after blunt trauma. *J Trauma* 2005; 59(5):1121–5.
19. Holmes JF, Akkinepalli R. Computed tomography versus plain radiography to screen for cervical spine injury: a meta-analysis. *J Trauma* 2005; 58(5):902–5.
20. Fabian TC, Patton JH Jr, Croce MA, et al. Blunt carotid injury. Importance of early diagnosis and anticoagulant therapy. *Ann Surg* 1996; 223:513–25.
21. Miller PR, Fabian TC, Bee TK, et al. Blunt cerebrovascular injuries: diagnosis and treatment. *J Trauma* 2001; 51:279–86.

22. Nederkoorn PJ, van der Graaf Y, HuninkMG. Duplex ultra-sound and magnetic resonance angiography compared with digital subtraction angiography in carotid artery stenosis: a systematic review. *Stroke* 2003; 34:1324–32.

23. Modrall JG, Weaver FA, Yellin AE. Diagnosis and management of penetrating vascular trauma and the injured extremity. *Emerg Med Clin N Am* 1998; 16(1):129–44.

24. Nassoura ZE, Ivatury RR, Simon RJ, et al. A reassessment of Doppler pressure indices in the detection of arterial lesions in proximity penetrating injuries of extremities: a prospective study. *Am J Emerg Med* 1996; 14(2):151–6.

25. Bungay HK, Berger J, Traill ZC, et al. Pneumothorax post CT-guided lung biopsy: a comparison between detection on chest radiographs and CT. *Br J Radiol* 1999; 72(864):1160–3.

26. Wolfman NT, Myers WS, Glauser SJ, Meredith JW, Chen MY. Validity of CT classification on management of occult Pneumothorax: a prospective study. *Am J Roentgenol* 1998; 171:1317–20.

27. Baumann MH, Strange C. The clinician's perspective on pneumothorax management. *Chest* 1997; 112(3):822–8.

28. Bottlang M, Simpson T, Sigg J, et al. Non-invasive reduction of open book pelvic fractures by circumferential compression. *J Ortho Trauma* 2002; 16(6):367–73.

29. Nagy KK, Joseph KT, Krosner SM, et al. The utility of head computed tomography after minimal head injury. *J Trauma* 1999; 46(2):268–70.

30. Livingston DH, Lavery RF, Passannante MR, et al. Emergency department discharge of patients with a negative cranial computed tomography scan after minimal head injury. *Ann Surg* 2000; 232(1):126–32.

31. Geijerstam JL, Britton M. Mild head injury: reliability of early computed tomographic findings in triage for admission. *Emerg Med J* 2005; 22:103–7.

32. Timsit JF, Farkas JC, Boyer JM, et al. Central vein catheter-related thrombosis in intensive care patients: incidence, risks factors, and relationship with catheter-related sepsis. *Chest* 1998; 114:207–13.

33. Merrer J, DeJonghe B, Golliot F, et al. Complications of femoral and subclavian venous catheterization in critically ill patients: a randomized controlled trial. *J Am Med Assoc* 2001; 286(6):700–7.

34. Hauswald M, Hsu M, Stockoff C: Maximising comfort and minimizing ischemia: a comparison of four methods of spinal immobilization. *Prehosp Emerg Care* 2000; 4(3):250–52.

35. Kwan I, Bunn F. Effects of prehospital spinal immobilization: a systematic review of randomized trials on healthy subjects. *Prehosp Disast Med* 2005; 20(1):47–53.

36. Black CA, Buderer NMF, Blaylock B, et al. Comparative study of risk factors for skin breakdown with cervical orthotic devices: Philadelphia and Aspen. *J Trauma Nurs* 1998; 5(3):62–66.

37. Kupas DF, Dula DJ, Pino BJ. Patient outcome using medical protocol to limit "lights and siren" transport. *Prehosp Disaster Med* 1994; 9(4):226–9.

38. Biggers WA, Zachariah BS, Pepe PE. Emergency medical vehicle collisions in an urban system. *Pre-hospital Disaster Med* 1996; 11(3):195–201.

39. Nathens AB, Maier RV, Brundage SI, et al. The effect of interfacility transfer on outcome in an urban trauma system. *J Trauma* 2003; 55(3):444–9.

40. Boque MC, Gualis B, Sandiumenge A, et al. Endotracheal tube intraluminal diameter narrowing after mechanical ventilation: use of acoustic reflectometry. *Intens Care Med* 2004; 30(12):2204–9.

41. Bijur PE, Kenny MK, Gallagher EJ. Intravenous morphine at 0.1 mg/kg is not effective for controlling severe acute pain in the majority of patients. *Ann Emerg Med* 2005; 46:362–67.

Chapter 8 | **Management of Infectious Diseases**

David J. Karras, Wayne A. Satz & Jeffrey Barrett

Introduction

The most common cause of death worldwide is infectious disease. Infections kill millions every year around the world, especially in third-world countries. But even in the most developed countries, infections are still a leading killer. Researchers' efforts to develop new ways to prevent infections, such as vaccination, and to treat infections, such as new antimicrobials, are constantly met with new obstacles. Increasing antibiotic resistance leading to new strains of common organisms, as well as the development of completely new types of infections. Methicillin-resistant *Staphylococcus aureus* (MRSA) and sepsis have recently gained significant attention in academic circles as well as the popular press; meanwhile, "old" infections such as pneumonia and meningitis continue to be leading causes of mortality in many populations. Emergency physicians must remain well informed about the trends and changing nature of infectious disease, while at the same time not ignoring the older diseases, in order to avoid the many pitfalls that are encountered in this field.

Pitfall | **Failure to consider acute bacterial endocarditis in febrile patients**

Infective endocarditis is relatively uncommon, but given the morbidity and mortality associated with a missed diagnosis it is important that emergency physicians consider the diagnosis to avoid the inappropriate discharge of patients with life-threatening infections. Furthermore, while infective endocarditis generally cannot be diagnosed in the emergency department (ED), the emergency physician often plays a critical role in obtaining initial blood cultures that are of vital importance in determining management. Failure to obtain necessary cultures may result long-term therapy that is unnecessarily protracted or even inappropriate.

The most common signs and symptoms of bacterial endocarditis are fever, malaise, night sweats, and a heart murmur, typically in a patient with underlying valvular heart disease [1]. The disease should be considered in any patient with an unexplained fever and a murmur. If evaluation for endocarditis is initiated in the ED or if hospitalization is warranted, three sets of blood cultures should be obtained from different sites over 1–2 h before initiating antimicrobial therapy. Careful skin prepping should be performed before drawing cultures to minimize the chances of contamination. Appropriately acquired cultures obtained in the ED may be the only opportunity for the pathogen and optimal therapy to be determined.

Pitfall | **Over-reliance on exam findings in acute bacterial endocarditis**

Fever is the most common manifestation of infective endocarditis, and is noted 90% of cases [2]. However, fever is a ubiquitous complaint among ED patients, and therefore is an exceedingly non-specific finding. Conversely, fever may be absent in the elderly, uremic, or debilitated patient with endocarditis, and should not be considered an essential component to the diagnosis [1].

> KEY FACT | **A murmur on initial presentation was only 35% sensitive for acute bacterial endocarditis … absence of a cardiac murmur, therefore, should not cause the emergency physician to exclude the diagnosis.**

Cardiac murmurs are often the physical finding that prompts the emergency physician to consider infectious endocarditis. Although the vast majority of patients with infectious endocarditis will develop a new murmur or change in character of a previously recognized murmur at some point in their illness, the finding will not necessarily be evident early in the course of the illness. In one series a murmur on initial presentation was only 35% sensitive for acute bacterial endocarditis [3]. Some specific populations are even less likely to have murmurs, including patients with right-sided valvular lesions and the elderly [4]. Absence of a cardiac murmur, therefore, should not cause the emergency physician to exclude the diagnosis of acute bacterial endocarditis if other features suggest the disease.

Other physical findings are associated with endocarditis. Roth spots are pale, ovoid retinal hemorrhages visible on fundoscopic exam. These are also seen in patients with anemia and collagen vascular disease, and are present in only about 5% with endocarditis [5]. Osler nodes are tender, indurated nodules on the palms of the hands and soles of the feet, and Janeway lesions are non-tender macules in the same areas. These lesions are more specific to infective endocarditis and should strongly suggest the diagnosis, but are insensitive and noted in <20% of cases [4]. Splinter hemorrhages of the nailbeds and mucosal petechaie are similarly insensitive and also non-specific, being found in leukemia, lymphoma, and uremia [2]. These findings can be very helpful when noted, but their absence should not dissuade the emergency physician from considering infective endocarditis as a diagnostic possibility.

Pitfall | Failure to consider endocarditis in intravenous drug users with neurological deficits

> KEY FACT | Neurologic complications occur in approximately one-third of cases of infective endocarditis.

Neurologic complications occur in approximately one-third of cases of infective endocarditis and typically present as a stroke syndrome. Valvular vegetations may embolize to the brain and causes cerebral infarction, usually in a branch of the middle cerebral artery, causing contralateral motor or sensory symptoms. However, infarction can occur anywhere in the cerebral circulation, producing a myriad of possible neurologic symptoms [2, 5].

Embolized infectious vegetations can impact at branch points in the cerebral vascular tree, causing the formation of mycotic aneurysms. These are noted in up to 2% of patients with infective endocarditis, causing symptoms due to mass effect, vascular leakage, or sudden rupture [5]. This can lead to a broad spectrum of clinical presentations ranging from subarachnoid hemorrhage to meningitis to coma. Infective endocarditis is therefore an important consideration when a young person who has no risk factors for premature cerebrovascular disease presents with stroke symptoms, particularly when the patient has risk factors for the development of infective endocarditis, such as intravenous drug use or valvular heart disease, or presents with a fever. Appropriate antimicrobial therapy, when promptly initiated, can reduce the rate of subsequent embolic events 10-fold [3, 5].

Pitfall | Misapplication of the pneumonia severity index

Community-acquired pneumonia (CAP) is very common, with over 5 million annual cases in the US. About 80% of cases can be appropriately managed as outpatients, and emergency physicians play a pivotal role in the management of this disease. The majority of patients with CAP remain on the antibiotic regimen started in the ED [6]. Furthermore, the emergency physician usually determines the treatment

setting – and will bear responsibility if a poor outcome ensues in an individual with CAP who is discharged to home.

In 1997, Fine and colleagues published a rule to predict the mortality associated with CAP in patients with specific co-morbidities, vital signs, and laboratory results [7]. Alternately known as the Pneumonia Severity Index (PSI), Patient Outcomes Research Trial (PORT) score, and the Fine rule, the algorithm is sometimes utilized to determine whether outpatient or inpatient therapy is appropriate for specific patients with CAP. Information immediately available upon ED presentation is used to determine whether patients with CAP meet Class I criteria (see Table 8.1): 50 years of age or younger, no history of congestive heart failure or neoplastic, cerebrovascular, renal, or liver disease, normal mental status, pulse <125/min, respiratory rate <30/min, systolic blood pressure >90 mmHg, and temperature between 35°C and 40°C. When all these criteria were met, CAP-related mortality was predicted to be 0.1% and outpatient therapy was considered appropriate.

Calculating CAP-related mortality in patients not meeting Class I criteria requires a complex point system based on 20 demographic, vital sign, and laboratory characteristics. Outpatient therapy was presumed to be suitable for patients assigned to Class II, who have a predicted mortality of 0.6%. A short-stay setting or home intravenous therapy might be appropriate for patients in Class III, with a predicted mortality of 0.9%. Patients in higher risk classes have predicted mortality of at least 9% and were obvious candidates for hospitalization.

> KEY FACT | Initial enthusiasm regarding use of the PSI to determine a patient's disposition has been tempered by some basic but important flaws in its design.

Initial enthusiasm regarding use of the PSI to determine a patient's disposition, however, has been tempered by some basic but important limitations in its design – the rule does not account for several factors that may have a significant impact on outcome. The index does not include immunocompromised individuals, and thus cannot be used in patients with HIV/AIDS, those undergoing treatment for malignancies, or others who are immunosuppressed. The study also excluded

Table 8.1 Low-risk ("Class I") criteria for patients with CAP.

Age ≤50 years
No prior history of congestive heart failure, neoplasm, cerebrovascular disease, renal disease, or liver disease
Normal mental status
Pulse <125/min
Respiratory rate <30/min
Systolic blood pressure >90 mmHg
Temperature between 35°C and 40°C

children and patients who had recently been hospitalized, and the rule cannot be applied to either of these groups.

The PSI algorithm also does not incorporate oxygen saturation. The PaO_2 enters into the equation only when its value is <60 mmHg. Most emergency physicians do not routinely obtain an arterial blood gas in patients with CAP unless the pulse oximetry value is low. It would be wise, therefore, to consider obtaining an arterial blood gas on any patient with CAP who is on the borderline between mortality risk classes, and certainly in any patient with a low pulse oximetry value. The result may make an important difference in disposition decision-making.

Another fundamental limitation of the PSI is its failure to incorporate social circumstances in the risk assessment. Homelessness and other unacceptable living arrangements, inability to obtain medication, absence of follow-up care, and inadequate social support may detrimentally affect the likelihood of successful outpatient therapy, but are not contained in the PSI algorithm. It is incumbent upon emergency physician to assess the intended outpatient treatment setting and, should it appear unsuitable for successful therapy, attempt to remedy deficiencies, involve social service workers, or simply override the PSI and admit the patient to the hospital.

In its revised treatment guidelines, the Infectious Disease Society of America (IDSA) urges physicians to use clinical judgment and consider the patient's overall health and social environment when making disposition decisions, rather than relying on the PSI alone [8]. This is important acknowledgment of the pitfalls inherent in blind application of decision rules. When the emergency physician rejects the PSI algorithm, medical decision-making should be documented to facilitate quality assurance reviews, reimbursement, and social service consultation.

Pitfall | Use of antibiotics for uncomplicated bronchitis

> KEY FACT | There is no evidence that the color, volume, or consistency of sputum predicts the presence of bacteria or need for antibiotics in acute uncomplicated bronchitis.

"Acute bronchitis" refers to a respiratory tract infection of <2–3 weeks' duration in which cough is a predominant feature and pneumonia has been excluded. Acute bronchitis in patients without underlying lung disease, immunocompromise, or co-morbidity is termed "acute uncomplicated bronchitis" and in 90% of cases is viral in etiology [9]. Placebo-controlled trials have failed to demonstrate a benefit to antibiotic therapy in the treatment of acute uncomplicated bronchitis, and meta-analyses demonstrate no salutary effect of antibiotics on duration of illness or lost work days. There is no evidence that the color, volume, or consistency of sputum predicts the presence of bacteria or need for antibiotics in

acute uncomplicated bronchitis. Furthermore, smokers without obstructive lung disease do not appear to benefit from routine administration of antibiotics for acute bronchitis.

Antimicrobials may be justified in patients with acute exacerbations of chronic bronchitis (AECB), which is usually considered to be an increase in sputum purulence, increase in sputum volume, or worsening dyspnea in a patient with chronic bronchitis. In contrast to acute uncomplicated bronchitis, AECB is associated with a bacterial respiratory infection in two-thirds of cases [10]. The presence of green sputum alone is a sensitive but fairly non-specific predictor of the presence of a bacterial pathogen [11]. A meta-analysis of nine comparable trials of antimicrobials in AECB favored antibiotic therapy by a small but statistically significant margin [12]. Most authorities agree that antibiotic therapy is appropriate for patients with moderate-to-severe cases of AECB and those with severe underlying lung disease [13]. There are multiple appropriate antibiotic options if therapy is warranted.

Pitfall | Inappropriate antibiotics prescription for sinusitis

Sinusitis is another heterogeneous disease with multiple etiologies and diagnostic uncertainties. In its broadest sense, sinusitis is an inflammation of the paranasal sinuses. Manifestations include nasal congestion, periorbital pain, purulent nasal discharge, maxillary toothache, fever, and percussion tenderness of the infected sinus. Acute sinusitis is a frequent complication of the common cold. These infections, representing the vast majority of acute sinusitis cases, are usually viral. Symptoms generally resolve within 10 days of onset, and antimicrobial therapy has no benefit.

Bacterial sinusitis usually results from superinfection of a pre-existing viral sinusitis. Unfortunately, no signs or symptoms of acute sinusitis – either individually or in combination – can reliably distinguish bacterial from viral infections. The "classic" findings of purulent nasal discharge, facial pain on bending forward, sinus tenderness, and maxillary toothache each identify only about half of patients with acute bacterial sinusitis, and are almost as frequently seen in patients with viral infections [14]. Fever is noted in only about a quarter of patients with bacterial sinusitis, but is far more suggestive of bacterial infection than the other signs. Plain sinus films have very little diagnostic utility: there are no findings on computed tomography (CT) that distinguish viral from bacterial infection, and sinus CT reveals a very high rate of abnormalities even in asymptomatic patients [15].

> KEY FACT | … classic signs of acute (bacterial) sinusitis: fever, marked pain, tenderness, or swelling in the sinus region, and molar pain without evidence of dental etiology.

Appropriate management of patients with acute sinusitis therefore relies on clinical criteria that are known to be unreliable. Most experts advise presuming that a bacterial infection is present in patients with multiple "classic" signs of acute sinusitis: fever, marked pain, tenderness, or swelling in the sinus region, and molar pain without evidence of dental etiology. It is important to remember that half of patients with even bacterial sinusitis will recover spontaneously within a week, though antimicrobial therapy may result in slightly faster recovery. It is therefore appropriate to prescribe antimicrobial therapy when there is reasonable suspicion that a bacterial infection is present based on the presence of "classic" signs [16] or in patients with protracted symptoms.

Patients lacking the "classic" signs of bacterial sinusitis usually have uncomplicated viral sinusitis, particularly when cold symptoms are present or patients complain of facial fullness, nasal obstruction, or cough. These individuals should generally not be offered antibiotics. However, when patients thought to have viral sinusitis show no symptom improvement after a week, it is reasonable to assume that they have developed a bacterial superinfection. This scenario occurs in about 2% of patients with uncomplicated viral sinusitis, and warrants antibiotic therapy [14]. Multiple treatment options are available for patients who warrant antibiotic therapy, and in most cases the antibiotic can be chosen on the basis of cost and convenience.

Pitfall | Routinely performing a CT before LP in patients with suspected meningitis

With the widespread availability of CT in the US it has become common practice to routinely image the brain before performing a lumbar puncture (LP) in evaluating ED patients suspected of having meningitis. A recent series found that three-fourths of patients with meningitis underwent a CT scan prior to LP [17]. More disturbingly, the majority of patients who undergo CT study prior to LP do not receive antibiotics before imaging is performed [18]. Delays related to obtaining CT imaging prior to LP performance and antibiotic administration result in 5-fold greater mortality among patients who are ultimately diagnosed with acute bacterial meningitis [19].

The true risk of LP resulting in uncal or cerebral herniation is widely overstated [20–22]. While all cases of purulent meningitis are associated with an increased intracranial pressure, herniation occurs in <1% of cases. Conversely, CT of the brain is normal in most cases of purulent meningitis, even among patients who subsequently herniate. CT findings that contraindicate LP are lateral shift of midline structures, loss of suprachiasmatic and basilar cisterns, obliteration of the fourth ventricle, or obliteration of the superior cerebellar and quadrigeminal plate cisterns with sparing of the ambient cisterns [23]. Abnormal findings that are not contraindications to LP include a new mass, stroke, or hemorrhage, absent signs of increased intracranial pressure. Using these criteria, a

Table 8.2 Historical and physical findings predicting the need for brain CT before LP.

Immunocompromised condition
Prior central nervous system disease
Seizure within prior 1 week
Cranial nerve deficits
Focal motor deficits
Depressed level of consciousness

recent study prospectively found that LP was contraindicated in <10% of patients with bacterial meningitis [24].

An important study by Hasbun and colleagues sets the standard of care in determining the need for CT study in patients with suspected meningtitis, and is cited by current meningitis treatment guidelines [25, 26]. In this prospective assessment of 301 adults with suspected meningitis, only 4% had CT findings that posed a risk of herniation, and each of these patients had significant historical or physical findings that reliably indicated the need for CT (Table 8.2). The historical findings were an immunocompromised state, previous central nervous system disease, or seizure within the previous week; physical findings were cranial nerve deficits, focal motor deficits, or a depressed level of consciousness (defined as the inability to answer two consecutive questions and follow two consecutive commands). While 3 patients with none of these findings had abnormal CT findings, all underwent LP without complication.

> KEY FACT | **The performance of brain CT should *never* delay appropriate treatment of patients with suspected bacterial meningitis.**

Interestingly, multiple studies have found papilledema not to be a useful clinical predictor of herniation [22, 27]. The finding may be absent in patients at significant risk for herniation, and conversely may be noted in those at minimal herniation risk. Papilledema may be difficult for the non-expert to detect, and appears to be an unreliable finding even under the best of circumstances. The takeaway points here are 2-fold: (1) brain CT should *not* be considered mandatory in every patient in whom meningitis is being evaluated, and (2) the performance of brain CT should *never* delay appropriate treatment of patients with suspected bacterial meningitis, as discussed below.

Pitfall | Delaying antibiotics in patients with suspected bacterial meningitis

Infectious disease guidelines recommend administering appropriate antibiotics to all patients with suspected meningitis within 30 min of presentation [25]. Despite these universal recommendations, recent studies continue to report significant delays in the administration of antibiotics [18, 25]. Administration of antimicrobials in an inpatient unit, rather than in the ED, is associated with a 5-h delay in medication delivery and a 3-fold increase in mortality [28]. A recent study reported that a delay >6 h between ED presentation and administration of antibiotics independently increased mortality in patients with bacterial meningitis by more than 8-fold [19]. Furthermore, timing of antibiotic administration was incrementally and closely related to mortality. It is important to note that many studies relating antibiotic administration to outcomes are confounded by factors that may have made early diagnosis of meningitis difficult.

> **KEY FACT** | Antibiotic administration does not appear to cause changes in cerebrospinal fluid (CSF) white blood cell, protein, or glucose levels … and does not change CSF Gram stain findings.

A common argument against immediate administration of antibiotics is that the practice may impair the diagnosis of bacterial meningitis on subsequent CSF testing. Antibiotic administration does not appear to cause changes in CSF white blood cell, protein, or glucose levels that would impede their diagnostic utility, and does not change CSF Gram stain findings [29, 30]. Almost all patients with acute bacterial meningitis still have diagnostic CSF abnormalities even if LP is delayed by 3 days. CSF cultures may be positive even after one dose of antibiotic administration, although the yield decreases with more fastidious organisms such as meningicoccus [31]. Importantly, other modalities can reliably identify the causative organism. Blood cultures obtained prior to antibiotic administration reveal the causative organism in 86% of patients with bacterial meningitis. Given the enormous mortality benefit associated with early administration of antibiotics, it is imperative to administer appropriate antimicrobial therapy as soon as bacterial meningitis is suspected.

Pitfall | **Failure to appreciate the range of CSF findings associated with bacterial meningitis**

The CSF white blood cell (WBC) count, protein, and glucose values are often unreliable tools for differentiating between viral and bacterial meningitis. Commonly accepted indicators of bacterial meningitis are total WBC count >5 cells/mm^3, polymorphonuclear WBC >75% of total WBC, CSF to serum glucose ratio <50%, and CSF protein >45 mg/dl [32]. WBC differentials may be misleading early in the course of meningitis, as more than 10% of patients with bacterial infection will have an initial lymphocytic predominance, and viral meningitis can be initially be dominated by neutrophils [30, 33, 34]. While each of these parameters is relatively insensitive, most authorities conclude that if any of these indices are abnormal, the incidence of bacterial meningitis is high enough to warrant presumptive diagnosis and aggressive treatment until culture results are available [18, 25, 30, 31, 35].

Pitfall | **Over-reliance on physical findings in diagnosing bacterial meningitis**

> **KEY FACT** | The classic findings of fever, nuchal rigidity, and altered mental status [were found] in less than half of patients with bacterial meningitis.

Failure to diagnose bacterial meningitis is in the top five malpractice claims in emergency medicine [36]. Virtually all patients with bacterial meningitis will have a fever, neck stiffness, headache, or altered mental status, and therefore the absence of all these findings can essentially exclude the diagnosis provided that the patient is capable of providing a relevant history [37]. Physical exam findings, however, are far less reliable. The largest prospective study to date noted the classic findings of fever, nuchal rigidity, and altered mental status in less than half of patients with bacterial meningitis, and a recent smaller study noted these classic findings in only 20% of cases [18].

Negative tests of nuchal rigidity, including the Kernig and Brudzinski signs, are commonly documented to indicate absence of meningitis. The Brudzinski sign refers to the patient's spontaneous flexion of the hips during attempts to passively flex the neck. The Kernig sign refers to the patient's reluctance to allow full extension of the knee when the hip is flexed 90°. Nuchal rigidity is more loosely defined, but is generally described as inability or discomfort during neck flexion. Each of these signs were developed and tested in patients with severe, late stage meningitis. While Kernig and Brudzinski signs are each about 95% specific for meningitis, their sensitivity is <10% [38]. Nuchal rigidity is slightly more sensitive, but less specific. Documenting the absence of meningeal signs, therefore, is not sufficient to exclude meningitis. Particularly in immunocompromised hosts, the presentation of meningitis is likely to be subacute, and negative exam findings are even more likely.

Jolt accentuation of headache may be a more sensitive maneuver for the diagnosis of meningitis. This test is performed by horizontally rotating the head two to three times per second; increased headache severity is considered a positive test. In a single small study, the maneuver displayed 97% sensitivity but only 60% specificity for the presence of meningitis [39].

Pitfall | **Failing to recognize methicillin-resistant *Staphylococcus aureus* as a common pathogen**

While MRSA emerged in the 1960s, until recently it has been associated only with patients exposed to antibiotics for extended periods of time or quartered in places harboring resistant pathogens. Traditional risk factors for MRSA included recent surgery or hospitalization, residence in a long-term care facility, prolonged antibiotic administration, hemodialysis, presence of indwelling devices or catheters, some chronic illnesses, and intravenous drug use. In 1998, a pediatric inpatient study made that made it clear that MRSA was relevant in patients with community-acquired infections [40]. While 87% of children hospitalized with MRSA infections between 1988 and 1990 had traditional risk factors for resistant infections, only 29% of patients with MRSA infections between 1993 and 1995 had such risk factors. The prevalence of MRSA infections in hospitalized children rose 25-fold in the 5 years between the study periods.

Subsequent reports have confirmed the importance of MRSA as a significant pathogen in a number of settings, including daycare, prisons, and among athletes [41–43]. A recent study of 1600 individuals with community-acquired MRSA infections found that 87% had skin or wound infections, but a small number had infections atypical for MRSA, including urinary tract infections, meningitis, osteomyelitis, sinusitis, and bacteremia [44]. Case reports have implicated MRSA in fatal cases of pneumonia in immunocompetent adults and children [45, 46] and in necrotizing fasciitis, a disease rarely associated with staphylococcal infections [47].

> KEY FACT | **Community-acquired MRSA is now a common and serious problem among ED patients … in a recent study of ED patients with skin infections, 59% were found to have MRSA.**

Community-acquired MRSA is now a common and serious problem among ED patients. In a recent multicenter study of 422 ED patients with skin infections, 59% were found to have MRSA [48]. All isolates were sensitive to trimethoprim-sulfamethoxazole, but only 90–95% were sensitive to clindamycin or tetracycline. A larger study of inpatients and outpatients found that infections were sensitive to vancomycin and 97% to trimethoprim-sulfamethoxazole, but only about 85% were sensitive to either clindamycin or tetracycline [44].

Despite the prevalence of MRSA skin lesions, antimicrobial therapy is not necessary for all ED patients with abscesses. Uncomplicated abscesses generally only require incision and drainage; antibiotics have not been shown to improve outcomes in these patients. Antibiotics are indicated for patients with abscesses complicated by cellulitis or fever, however,

and the selected agent should be active against MRSA. Trimethoprim-sulfamethoxizole is an effective and inexpensive option. Patients allergic to sulfa may be offered clindamycin or tetracycline, but it should be recognized that a significant number of organisms have developed resistance to these antibiotics. Linezolid is another option, but a course of therapy costs over $1000. Some authorities advise adding rifampin to a course of trimethoprim-sulfamethoxizole to improve efficacy [49]. Furthermore, it has been noted that unlike abscesses, cellulitis is more commonly due to *Streptococcus pyogenes* than to *Staphylococcus aureus*, and trimethoprim-sulfamethoxizole may be less effective for these infections. Some experts therefore advise that patients who have cellulitis without abscess be treated with a combination of a first-generation cephalosporin and trimethoprim-sulfamethoxizole, or with clindamycin alone [49].

Pitfall | **Failure to aggressively treat sepsis**

> KEY FACT | **Severe sepsis (carries) an estimated mortality rate of 27% – killing as many people annually as acute myocardial infarction.**

Emergency physicians frequently encounter sepsis, in widely varying degrees of severity. Sepsis is broadly defined as the presence of at least two components of the systemic inflammatory response syndrome (SIRS) and a suspected source of infection (see Table 8.3). When associated with organ dysfunction it is termed "severe sepsis," while "septic shock" is associated with hypotension unresponsive to intravenous fluid resuscitation without another cause for hypotension [50]. A recent analysis determined that there are 751,000 cases of severe sepsis annually in the US, carrying an estimated mortality rate of 27% – killing as many people annually as acute myocardial infarction [51]. Although septic shock is not usually a diagnostic dilemma, subtle manifestations of organ dysfunction or tissue hypoxia can be difficult to appreciate without frank hypotension.

> KEY FACT | **Early, goal-directed therapy of patients … significantly decreased in-hospital mortality from 47% to 31%.**

In a 2001 study, Rivers et al. showed that early, goal-directed therapy (EGDT) of patients with severe sepsis and septic shock significantly decreased in-hospital mortality from 47% to 31% [52]. This approach to resuscitation targets the normalization of central venous oxygen saturation instead of the traditional target of blood pressure normalization. The goals of EGDT during the initial resuscitation period (first 6 h) include maintenance of the central venous

Table 8.3 Definitions of sepsis states [50].

Components of SIRS. SIRS is present when at least two criteria are present	
Temperature <36°C or >38°C	
Pulse >90 beats/min	
Respiratory rate >20 breaths/min or PaCO$_2$ <32 mmHg	
WBC <4 k or >12 k	
Sepsis syndromes	
Sepsis	SIRS associated with an infection, proven or suspected
Severe sepsis	Sepsis associated with organ dysfunction
Septic shock	Sepsis associated with hypotension despite adequate volume resuscitation

Table 8.4 Initial resuscitation goals in patients with sepsis.

Central venous pressure 8–12 mmHg
Mean arterial pressure ≥65 mmHg
Central venous (superior vena cava) or mixed venous oxygen saturation ≥70%
Urine output ≥0.5 ml/kg/h

pressure between 8 and 12 mmHg, mean arterial pressure ≥65 mmHg, central venous (superior vena cava) or mixed venous oxygen saturation ≥70%, and urine output ≥0.5 ml/kg/h (see Table 8.4). If fluid resuscitation is accomplished with a resulting central venous pressure of 8–12 mmHg, but the central venous oxygen saturation or mixed venous oxygen saturation remains <70%, then a dobutamine infusion should be administered to accomplish the goal. If the patient's hematocrit is <30%, packed red blood cells should be transfused to a goal of ≥30% prior to or during the dobutamine infusion.

A post hoc analysis of this data showed that EGDT made an even more dramatic difference in normotensive patients with elevated serum lactate levels (>4 mmol/l), dropping mortality at 60 days from 70% to 24% [53]. Nguyen et al. also showed that failure to improve an elevated lactate level during the initial resuscitation of patients with severe sepsis more than doubled mortality [54]. These data suggest that microcirculatory defects causing global tissue hypoxia may exist without frank hypotension, and that correction of this dysfunction may reverse the process before organ failure and death ensues.

Pitfall | **Failure to ensure adequate antimicrobial treatment in severe sepsis and septic shock**

It seems intuitive that adequately treating patients with severe sepsis or septic shock entails using antibiotics that are effective against the infecting microorganism and initiating therapy as quickly as possible. In fact, recent guidelines for the management of severe sepsis and septic shock call for the administration of intravenous antibiotics within 1 h of recognizing the syndrome [55]. What may not be readily apparent is the impact on outcome that inappropriate antibiotic therapy may have, or how frequently an error in coverage is made. A recent study found that 15% of patients with sepsis received antibiotics ineffective against the infecting microorganism. While the effect on mortality was most pronounced in those with septic shock, it was significant in all patients. In patients with septic shock, inappropriate antibiotic treatment doubled 14-day mortality from 40 to 80% [56]. The practicing emergency physician should be aware of the importance of antimicrobial efficacy when treating sepsis, and cover broadly when the source is unclear.

Pearls for Improving Patient Outcomes

- Do not discount the diagnosis of bacterial endocarditis based simply on the absence of a murmur.
- The disposition of patients with pneumonia should be based primarily on the physician's clinical judgement and not purely on the PSI or other such decision instruments.
- Avoid prescribing antibiotics in all cases of bronchitis and sinusitis. Consider the patient co-morbidities and disease severity before dispensing antibiotics.
- Use of brain CT before all LPs is unnecessary and often results in delays in care of the patient. Never delay antibiotics while awaiting the CT in patients with suspected bacterial meningitis.
- Do not withhold antibiotics in patients with suspected bacterial meningitis out of fear of impairing the CSF analysis. CSF results remain diagnostic even after antibiotic administration.
- Antibiotic regimens for community-acquired cellulitis should include coverage for MRSA in many ED populations now.
- Severe sepsis and septic shock must be treated aggressively. EGDT and broad-spectrum antibiotics can significantly decrease mortality in these patients.

References

1. Mylonakis E, Calderwood SB. Infective endocarditis in adults. *New Eng J Med* 2001; 345(16):1318–30.
2. Crawford MH, Durack DT. Clinical presentation of infective endocarditis. *Cardiol Clin* 2003; 21:159–66.
3. Saccent M, Cobbs CG. Clinical approach to infective endocarditis. *Cardiol Clin* 1996; 14(3):352–62.
4. Cunha BA, Gill MV, Lazar JM. Acute infective endocarditis: diagnostic and therapeutic approach. *Inf Dis Clin N Am* 1996; 10:811–31.
5. Kaye AR. Neurologic complications of infective endocarditis. *Neurol Clin* 1993; 11:419–37.
6. Marrie TJ. Community-acquired pneumonia: epidemiology, etiology, treatment. *Infect Dis Clin N Am* 1998; 12:723–40.
7. Fine MJ, Auble TE, Yealy DM, et al. A prediction rule to identify low-risk patients with community-acquired pneumonia. *New Engl J Med* 1997; 336:243–50.

8. Mandell LA, Bartlett JG, Dowell SF, et al. Update of practice guidelines or the management of community-acquired pneumonia in immunocompetent adults. *Clin Infect Dis* 2003; 37: 1405–33.

9. Gonzales R, Bartlett JG, Besser RE, et al. Principles of appropriate antibiotic use for treatment of uncomplicated acute bronchitis: background. *Ann Emerg Med* 2001; 37:720–7.

10. Sethi S. Infectious exacerbations of chronic bronchitis: diagnosis and management. *J Antimicr Chemother* 1999; 43:A97–105.

11. Stockley RA, O'Brien C, Pye A, Hill SL. Relationship of sputum color to nature and outpatient management of COPD. *Chest* 2000; 117:1638–45.

12. Saint S. Antibiotics in chronic obstructive pulmonary disease: a meta-analysis. *J Am Med Assoc* 1995; 273:957–60.

13. Grossman RF. Guidelines for the treatment of acute exacerbations of chronic bronchitis. *Chest* 1997; 112:110–15.

14. Picirillo JF. Acute bacterial sinusitis. *New Engl J Med* 2004; 351:902–10.

15. Gwaltney JM, Phillips CD, Miller RD, Riker DK. Computed tomographic study of the common cold. *New Engl J Med* 2004: 330:25–30.

16. Snow V, Mottur-Pilson C, Hickner JM. Principles of appropriate antibiotic use for acute sinusitis in adults. *Ann Intern Med* 2001; 134:495–7.

17. Durand ML, Calderwood SB, Weber DJ, et al. Acute bacterial meningitis: a review of 493 episodes. *New Engl J Med* 1993; 328:21–8.

18. van de Beek D, de Gans J, Spanjaard L, et al. Clinical features and prognostic factors in adults with bacterial meningitis. *New Engl J Med* 2004; 351:1849.

19. Proulx N, Fréchette D. Delays in the administration of antibiotics are associated with mortality from adult acute bacterial meningitis. *Q J Med* 2005; 98(4):291–8.

20. Haslam RH. Role of computerized tomography in the early management of bacterial meningitis. *J Pediatr* 1991; 119:157–9.

21. Richards PG, Towu-Aghanste E. Dangers of lumbar puncture. *Br Med J* 1986; 292:605–6.

22. Duffy GP. Lumbar puncture in the presence of raised intracranial pressure. *Br Med J* 1969; 1:407–9.

23. Gower DJ, Baker AL, Bell WO, Ball MR. Contraindications to lumbar puncture as defined by computed cranial tomography. *J Neurol Neurosurg Psychiatry* 1987; 50:1071–4.

24. Gopal AK, Whitehouse JD, Simel DL, Corey GR. Cranial computed tomography before lumbar puncture: a prospective clinical evaluation. *Arch Intern Med* 1999; 159:2681–5.

25. Hasbun R, Abrahams J, Jekel J, Quagliarello VJ. Computed tomography of the head before lumbar puncture in adults with suspected meningitis. *New Engl J Med* 2001; 345:1727–33.

26. Tunkel AR, Hartman BJ, Kaplan SL, et al. Practice guidelines for the management of bacterial meningitis. *Clin Infect Dis* 2004; 39:1267.

27. Sharp CG, Steinhart CM. Lumbar puncture in the presence of increased intracranial pressure: the real danger. *Pediatr Emerg Care* 1987; 3:39–43.

28. Miner JR, Heegaard W, Mapes A, Biros M. Presentation, time to antibiotics, and mortality of patients with bacterial meningitis at an urban county medical center. *J Emerg Med* 2001; 21:387–92.

29. Blazer S, Berant M, Alon U. Bacterial meningitis. Effect of antibiotic treatment on cerebrospinal fluid. *Am J Clin Pathol* 1983; 80:386–7.

30. Talan DA, Zibulewsky. Relationship of clinical presentation to time to antibiotics for the emergency department management of suspected bacterial meningitis. *Ann Emerg Med* 1993; 22:1733–8.

31. Coant PN, Kornberg AE, Duffy LC, Dryja DM, Hassan SM. Blood culture results as determinants in the organism identification of bacterial meningitis. *Pediatr Emerg Care* 1992; 8:200–5.

32. Seehusen DA, Reeves MM. Cerebrospinal fluid analysis. *Am Fam Pract* 2003; 68:6.

33. Spach DH, Jackson LA. Central nervous system infections. *Neurol Clin* 1999; 17:711–35.

34. Bonsu BK, Harper MB. Accuracy and test characteristics of cerebral spinal fluid for predicting meningitis in children with low white blood cell counts in cerebral spinal fluid. *Acad Emerg Med* 2005; 12(4):303–9

35. McMillan DA, Lin CY, Aronin SI, Quagliarello VJ. Community-acquired bacterial meningitis in adults: categorization of causes and timing of death. *Clin Infect Dis* 2001; 33:969–75.

36. Selbst SM, Friedman MJ. Epidemiology and etiology of malpractice lawsuits involving children in US emergency departments and urgent care centers. *Pediatr Emerg Care* 2005; 21:165–9.

37. Attia J, Hatala R, Cook DJ, Wong JG. The rational clinical examination: does this adult patient have acute meningitis? *J Am Med Assoc* 1999; 282:175.

38. Thomas KE, Hasbun R, Jekel J, Quagliarello VJ. The diagnostic accuracy of Kernig's sign, Brudzinski's sign, and nuchal rigidity in adults with suspected meningitis. *Clin Infect Dis* 2002; 35:46.

39. Uchihara T, Tsukagoshi H. Jolt accentuation of headache: the most sensitive sign of CSF pleocytosis. *Headache* 1991; 31:167.

40. Herold BC, Immergluck LC, Maranan MC, et al. Community-acquired methicillin-resistant *Staphylococcus aureus* in children with no identified predisposing risk. *J Am Med Assoc* 1998; 279:593–8.

41. CDC. Methicillin-resistant *Staphylococcus aureus* infections in correctional facilities – Georgia, California, and Texas, 2001–2003. *MMWR* 2003; 52:992–5.

42. CDC. Methicillin-resistant *Staphylococcus aureus* infections among competitive sports participants, 2000–2003. *MMWR* 2003; 52:992–6.

43. Kazakova SV, Hageman JC, Matava M, et al. A clone of methicillin-resistant *Staphylococcus aureus* among professional football players. *New Engl J Med* 2005; 352:468–75.

44. Fridkin SK, Hageman JC, Morrison M, et al. Methicillin-resistant *Staphylococcus aureus* disease in three communities. *New Engl J Med* 2005; 352:1436–44.

45. Gillet Y, Issartel B, Vanhems P, et al. Association between *Staphylococcus aureus* strains carrying gene for Panton-Valentine leukocidin and highly lethal necrotising pneumonia in young immunocompetent patients. *Lancet* 2002; 359:753–9.

46. Frazee BW, Salz TO, Lambert L, Perdreau-Remington F. Fatal community-associated methicillin-resistant *Staphylococcus aureus* pneumonia in an immunocompetent young adult. *Ann Emerg Med* 2005; 46:401–4.

47. Miller LG, Perdreau-Remington F, Rieg G, et al. Necrotizing fasciitis caused by community-associated methicillin-resistant *Staphylococcus aureus* in Los Angeles. *New Engl J Med* 2005; 352:1445–53.

48. Moran GJ, Krishnadasan A, Gorwitz RJ, et al. Methicillin-resistant *S. aureus* infections among patients in emergency department. *New England Journal of Medicine* 2006; 355:666–74.

49. Moran GJ, Talan DA. Community-associated methicillin-resistant *Staphylococcus aureus*: is it in your community and should it change practice? *Ann Emerg Med* 2005; 45:321–2.

50. Levy MM, Fink MP, Marschall JC, et al. 2001 SCCM/ ESICM/ ACCP/ATS/SIS International sepsis definitions conference. *Crit Care Med* 2003; 31:1250–6.

51. Angus DC, Linde-Zwirble WT, Lidicker J, et al. Epidemiology of severe sepsis in the United States: analysis of incidence, outcome, and associated costs of care. *Crit Care Med* 2001; 29:1303–10.

52. Rivers E, Nguyen B, Havstad S, et al. Early goal-directed therapy in the treatment of severe sepsis and septic shock. *New Engl J Med* 2001; 345:1368–77.

53. Donnino MW, Nguyen B, Jacobsen G, et al. Cryptic septic shock: a sub-analysis of early, goal-directed therapy. *Chest* 2003; 124(4):90S.

54. Nguyen HB, Rivers EP, Knoblich BP, et al. Early lactate clearance is associated with improved outcome in severe sepsis and septic shock. *Crit Care Med* 2004; 32:1637–42.

55. Dellinger RP, Carlet JM, Masur H, et al. Surviving sepsis campaign guidelines for the management of severe sepsis and septic shock. *Crit Care Med* 2004; 32:858–73.

56. Valles J, Rello J, Ochangavia A, et al. Community-acquired bloodstream infection in critically Ill adult patients – impact of shock and inappropriate antibiotic activity on survival. *Chest* 2003; 123:1615–24.

Chapter 9 | **Wound Care in Emergency Medicine**

Siamak Moayedi & Mercedes Torres

Introduction

Emergency physicians are the primary providers of post-traumatic wound management. Over 11 million traumatic wounds are managed in emergency departments (ED) in the US annually [1]. Of these, over 50% occur as a result of blunt trauma, while the remainder involve the penetration of sharp objects, such as metal, glass, or wood. The majority of these wounds occur on patients' heads and upper extremities, both highly visible areas [2]. As a result, the cosmetic appearance of healed wounds is a priority for both patients and emergency physicians. According to a survey of ED patients, the top four concerns of patients with a laceration include the cosmetic appearance, preservation of function, decreasing the pain of the repair, and avoiding a wound infection [3]. As these key outcomes are closely related to the specific wound care techniques used during the initial ED encounter, it is of utmost importance that emergency physicians stay abreast of the biggest pitfalls in wound care in order to avoid negative outcomes. A national survey of wound care techniques revealed that many practitioners manage wounds in ways that are contrary to the recommendations of published literature [4]. Furthermore, between 5% and 20% of all emergency physician malpractice claims involve issues of wound care, with up to 11% of all malpractice dollars being awarded for these cases [2]. These data further emphasize the importance of recognizing and avoiding many of the common pitfalls of wound care reviewed in the subsequent sections.

Pitfall | **Failure to properly prepare a wound prior to closure**

Beyond anesthesia, inspection, and evaluation for foreign body, proper preparation of a wound improves its outcome. Despite available evidence-based recommendations, many practitioners continue to employ techniques and utilize products that are unnecessary, and in some cases detrimental. In a survey distributed to predominantly board certified emergency physicians, investigators found that despite the existence of wound management guidelines, 90% of physicians treated wounds based on personal preference. Thirty-eight percent soaked wounds, 67% scrubbed wounds, 27% irrigated wounds with inadequate technique, and 21% used concentrated povidone–iodine solution or hydrogen peroxide [4].

> KEY FACT | **The necessary pressure for wound irrigation can be accomplished by pushing fluid in a 30–60 ml syringe through a 19-gauge catheter.**

Wound irrigation with high pressure and adequate volume has been shown to have a dramatic impact on wound infection rates. Simply soaking a wound provides no advantage and may be detrimental to its ultimate outcome [2]. The necessary pressure for wound irrigation can be accomplished by pushing fluid in a 30–60 ml syringe through a 19-gauge catheter. This is a highly effective means of reducing potentially infective material from a wound [5, 6]. The pressure generated through this technique cannot be reproduced by puncturing containers of irrigation fluid and squeezing with maximal hand pressure [1]. The data regarding the volume of irrigation fluid necessary is limited. Most authorities recommend 50–100 ml of irrigation fluid per cm of laceration. However, these sources agree that the volume of irrigation should be adjusted to the wound characteristics and degree of contamination [2, 7]. For instance, a contaminated scalp wound may require less irrigation solution than an extremity wound.

Irrigation of highly vascularized structures such as the face and scalp may not be as critical. Hollander et al. demonstrated that not irrigating clean-appearing, simple facial and scalp lacerations did not alter the rates of infection [8]. In addition, at very high irrigation pressures, research suggests that infection rates may actually increase due to tissue damage. Therefore, care must be taken not to use high-pressure irrigation in vascular wounds with loose alveolar tissue [7].

The choice of irrigation solution can have significant effects on wound healing. Antiseptic solutions such as chlorhexidine, povidone–iodine 10% solution, hydrogen peroxide, and detergents are toxic to tissues and impede wound healing [9, 10]. Studies comparing diluted 1% povidone–iodine to normal saline have not shown any difference in infection rates [11]. Furthermore, given the prevalence of iodine sensitivity, the use of diluted iodine irrigation is discouraged. More recently, published studies have concluded that there is no clinically significant difference in infection rates between simple wounds irrigated with potable tap water and sterile normal saline [12, 13].

Another misguided practice which has been shown to increase infection rates is shaving the area surrounding a wound prior to repair [14, 15]. If hair removal is required for adequate access to or visualization of a wound, it is recommended that the hair is clipped, rather than shaved, at the skin level [16]. One effective alternative is to use petroleum products to comb hair away from the wound. Care must be taken to remove small pieces of hair from the wound prior to closure.

Finally, many practitioners routinely use sterile gloves for the repair of simple lacerations. Studies supporting this practice are lacking. In a prospective study of 816 patients with simple wounds randomized to wound repaired using sterile versus clean gloves, there was no difference in subsequent infection rates [17].

Pitfall | **Failure to detect the presence of a foreign body in a wound**

> KEY FACT | **Missed retained foreign bodies are the fifth leading cause of malpractice claims against emergency physicians in the US [1].**

When unrecognized, retained foreign bodies can cause significant morbidity, including local inflammation, infection, and compression of vital structures [18]. Emergency physicians have a variety of tools at their disposal to assist with the detection of foreign bodies. The key to addressing a foreign body is finding it.

Detection of foreign bodies by clinical examination alone has proven unreliable. If the bottom of a wound is visible and no foreign body is seen, 7% of subsequent X-rays have been shown to be positive for the presence of a foreign body (see Figure 9.1). Furthermore, when the bottom of a wound is not visualized, clinically undetected foreign bodies have been found on X-rays in 21% of cases [1]. There are clinical clues that can raise suspicion for the presence of a foreign body:

Persistent pain
Drainage from wound
Palpable mass at wound site
Surface discoloration
Blood-stained wound tract
History of contact with broken glass
Clenched-fist injury
Puncture wounds
Motor vehicle accident
Foreign body sensation by patient

These include persistent pain, drainage, a palpable mass, surface discoloration, or a blood-stained tract. Obtaining a history of glass breaking while in contact with the skin, blunt trauma with tooth fragments, clenched-fist injuries, puncture

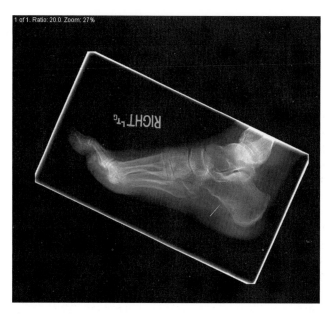

Figure 9.1 Plain radiograph demonstrating metallic foreign body in the foot.

wounds, motor vehicle accidents, and foreign body sensation should raise suspicion for retained foreign bodies in a wound [18]. According to a study of wounds caused by glass, 15% had retained glass within the wound. Patients reporting foreign body sensation had a positive predictive value of 31% and a negative predictive value of 89%. However, using patient perception alone to determine X-ray eligibility would have missed 57% of wounds with retained glass [19].

One of the primary diagnostic modalities used for detection of foreign bodies in wounds is X-ray. Legal precedents have shown that practitioners who failed to X-ray wounds caused by glass were unsuccessful in defending themselves in 60% of cases [1]. Radio opaque foreign bodies include glass, metal, bone, teeth, pencil graphite, certain plastics, gravel, some aluminum, and some sand [2, 18]. X-rays can detect greater than 50% of glass with a single dimension between 0.5 and 2.0 mm, and virtually all with a dimension greater than 2.0 mm [1, 7, 18]. Underpenetrated X-rays, highlighting the soft tissues are more useful for detecting retained foreign bodies not visualized with standard X-rays [18, 20]. In addition, it is possible to visualize a filling defect on a soft tissue X-ray created by a radiolucent foreign body [20]. One problem with X-rays is their two-dimensional quality. If detected, it is often difficult to determine the exact location of the foreign body and its spatial relation to other vital structures. Obtaining multiple views and using markers such as paper clips or needles can assist with localization of the foreign body using X-ray alone [18].

When suspicion is high for a radiolucent foreign body, or a foreign body in close proximity to vital structures, a computed tomography (CT) scan is often the study of choice. CTs are useful for detecting radiolucent objects such as wood, certain plastics, thorns, and spines. In addition, they can detect the presence of vegetative material, which has a high rate of infection and inflammatory complication. This benefit is optimized within the first 48 hours because vegetative foreign bodies absorb water within tissues, changing their density to appear very similar to soft tissue, and therefore more difficult to differentiate [1]. Regardless the age of a wound, CTs are still 100 times more sensitive for detecting various densities of objects as compared with X-ray. In addition, they provide a visualization of the location of foreign bodies in relation to surrounding structures [18]. The ability to localize a foreign body assists the practitioner in deciding whether it should be removed and if removal should be surgical. Magnetic resonance imaging (MRI) has also been shown to be useful in identifying retained vegetative matter, but cannot be used if there is any suspicion for metal or gravel foreign bodies. The cost and "inconvenience" of MRI has excluded this as a primary imaging modality for the detection of retained wound foreign bodies [18].

Another diagnostic modality that has been shown to be efficient and less costly is bedside ultrasound. The value of ultrasound in detecting and localizing wound foreign bodies is dependent upon the provider's skill and the size of the object. A 7.5 MHz linear probe is optimal for wound examination, allowing approximately 3 cm of tissue penetration. The technique involves rotating the probe in a perpendicular position to the skin in order to attempt to localize the foreign body in cross section [21]. Increasing the frequency of the probe improves its ability to detect smaller foreign bodies [22]. One recent study examining the utility of bedside ultrasound in the detection of wood foreign bodies demonstrated a sensitivity of 95% and specificity of 89% [23]. Others have cited ranges of sensitivity from 50% to 90%, and specificity from 70% to 97%. Certain types of foreign bodies have characteristic appearances on ultrasound. Metal or glass is described as having a comet-tail appearance, while wood, plastic, sand, and pebbles often demonstrate acoustic shadowing similar to that seen with gallstones [21]. Unlink CT scans, ultrasound may be more helpful when patients present greater than 48 hours after suffering their wound, as the inflammation around a foreign body makes it easier to identify its location [23]. However, the use of bedside ultrasound is complicated by false positives. These include echo artifacts that can be made by air pockets, calcifications, old scar tissue, blood, sutures, sesamoid bones, or purulence [18]. In addition, the presence of multiple tissue planes can complicate ultrasound guided localization [24]. Once a foreign body is located, ultrasound can provide real-time visualization of its removal as well as identifying other smaller surrounding foreign bodies [25].

Pitfall | Failure to recognize the morbidity associated with plantar puncture wounds

Plantar puncture wounds represent a unique challenge for physicians. The soles of the feet are the most common site of puncture wounds in the lower extremities. The force of a patient's weight onto a foreign body and the relative small distance from the skin to highly susceptible structures such as bones and joints make this injury especially prone to infection and significant morbidity. Care of the patient presenting with an acute plantar puncture remains controversial. The two most controversial areas involve the extent of wound exploration/debridement and the question of antibiotic prophylaxis.

Many authors have asserted that plantar punctures have a high predilection for retained foreign bodies. Schwab and Powers reported a 3% rate of retained foreign body after initial surface cleansing without wound exploration [26]. A larger study of 887 patients also reported a 3% incidence of foreign body retention. Half of these were pieces of foot wear, while the remainder included rust and dirt [27]. However, because many patients with this injury do not present to the ED unless they experience continued pain or infection, the true incidence of retained foreign body may be lower [28].

There are no prospective, randomized trials that demonstrate the utility of prophylactic antibiotics in these injuries. One of the most quoted studies recommending antibiotic prophylaxis was an uncontrolled, observational study, with optional use of antibiotics [29]. Most authorities defer to the individual clinician regarding the use of antibiotics with the caveat that antibiotics do not compensate for inadequate wound care [18].

> KEY FACT | **High-risk wound which may require aggressive debridement include injuries through rubber-soled shoes, injuries over metatarsal phalangeal joints, and injuries in patients with high-risk comorbidities.**

Uncomplicated puncture wounds without concern for retained foreign bodies may not require any wound exploration, but close follow up is advised [26]. Many aggressive and time-consuming procedures, such as coring and wound extension, have been described for the evaluation of these wounds. Coring refers to excision of a block of tissue down to the subcutaneous layer to allow visualization and access to foreign bodies and contaminated tissue. There is no definitive study showing that routinely coring puncture wounds reduces the incidence of infection. Furthermore, extensive debridement and coring may actually delay wound healing and cause undue pain [18]. Authors have argued that high-risk wounds which may require aggressive debridement include injuries through rubber-soled shoes, injuries over metatarsal phalangeal joints, and injuries in patients with high-risk comorbidities, such as diabetes and neuropathy [2].

> KEY FACT | **The rate of osteomyelitis caused by plantar puncture wounds is between 0.04% and 2%.**

A concerning clinical scenario involves a previous puncture wound presenting days later with evidence of infection. Delayed presentation is a significant marker for deep-seated infection [30]. These cases should prompt a thorough investigation for a retained foreign body [18]. Referral to specialists for removal of all but superficial foreign bodies and aggressive debridement is recommended. A high level of concern for osteomyelitis is raised when a wound relapses or fails to respond to the initial therapy. Overall, the rate of osteomyelitis caused by plantar puncture wounds is between 0.04% and 2% [18]. Advanced imaging techniques such as MRI may be required for diagnosis.

Although gram-positive organisms remain the most common cause of infection, several studies have demonstrated the role of *Pseudomonas aeruginosa* when the puncture occurs through rubber-soled foot wear [7]. It is presumed that the moist inner sole of the shoe provides a suitable environment for this bacterium [31]. When considering antibiotic prophylaxis, ciprofloxacin is still the antibiotic of choice. The newer quinolones, despite demonstrating better efficacy against gram-positive organisms, are less effective against Pseudomonas.

Pitfall | **Indiscriminate use of prophylactic antibiotics for bite wounds**

> KEY FACT | **Studies of infection rates after mammalian bites have failed to demonstrate any significant difference between those who received prophylactic antibiotics and those who received placebo except in cases of high-risk wounds.**

On a yearly basis, several million people are bitten by mammals in the USA. Almost one half of all children in the USA will be bitten by a dog at some point during their childhood [32]. A small proportion of adults and children with bite wounds, somewhere between 1 and 2 million, seek treatment. Animal bites comprise 1% of all ED visits annually, with dog bites accounting for 80% of those visits [2, 33, 34]. Although bite wounds are a commonly encountered complaint among emergency physicians, their management remains controversial. They are thought to be at increased risk for infections and wound complications, leading to the recommended use of prophylactic antibiotics. However, studies of infection rates after mammalian bites have failed to demonstrate any significant difference between those who received prophylactic antibiotics and those who received placebo except in cases of high-risk wounds [7, 32, 35, 36].

One of the primary concerns with any bite wound is possible inoculation of the soft tissue with oral flora. The specific organisms of concern vary based on the type of mammal which has bitten the patient. While over 80% of animal bites reported are from dogs, only 4–25% of these become infected.

Cat bites, although less frequent, are more commonly complicated by infection rates that range between 30% and 80%, depending on the study referenced [34, 37]. Human bites are considered to have the highest risk of infection when compared with dogs and cats. Although most bite wound infections contain mixed flora, pasturella is the primary culprit in both dog and cat bite wounds. Pasturella causes a rapid onset of signs and symptoms of infection, typically within 24 hours of the initial injury [37]. Streptococci, Staphylococci, Moraxella, Corynebacterium, and Neisseria are the next most common pathogens cultured from animal bite wounds. Infections attributed to Staphylococci and Streptococci typically manifest as nonpurulent wounds with lymphangitis. In addition to the aforementioned flora, over 50% of bite wounds contain anaerobic organisms [37, 38]. Therefore, optimal prophylactic agents would include beta lactams with a beta lactamase inhibitor, second-generation cephalosporins with anaerobic activity, or a combination of clindamycin and a fluoroquinolone. Traditional choices such as first-generation cephalosporins, ampicillin, or penicillin alone, have proven ineffective and are not recommended [37].

Although there is evidence that bite wounds in general have higher infection rates as compared with other types of wounds, the utility of prophylactic antibiotics for all bite wounds has been questioned. According to a 2005 Cochrane Database review of eight randomized controlled trials, prophylactic antibiotics were associated with a statistically significant reduction in the rate of infections after human bites, but not after cat or dog bites [32]. However, other studies suggest that even human bite wounds that involve minor injuries have not been shown to benefit from prophylactic antibiotics [36]. Thus, physicians must consider more than just the species of the biting mammal when evaluating the benefit of prophylactic antibiotics. It is safer and more cost-effective to reserve prophylactic antibiotics for high-risk wounds and high-risk patients (Table 9.1).

Focusing on the characteristics of the wound, deep puncture wounds, wounds with extensive crush injury or devitalized tissue, and wounds involving underlying muscle or tendons are at higher risk of infection. In addition, any wound involving an underlying bone fracture, retained foreign body, or joint should be considered an increased infection risk [2].

Table 9.1 Wound and patient characteristics that increase the risk of wound infection.

Wound characteristics
    Deep punctures
    Wounds with extensive crush injury or devitalized tissue
    Underlying muscle or tendon involvement
Patient characteristics
    Diabetes
    Immunocompromised state
    History of endocarditis
    Presence of orthopedic prostheses

Bites on the hand, including fight bites, maintain a particularly high risk of infection and current evidence supports the use of prophylactic antibiotics in these cases [32].

> **KEY FACT** | Patients who present greater than 72 hours after the initial bite with no signs of infection do not require antibiotic prophylaxis.

Patient-specific factors which would support the use of prophylactic antibiotics include a history of diabetes mellitus, immunocompromise, endocarditis, and orthopedic prostheses. The time between the bite and presentation to the ED is another important factor in determining the value of antibiotic prophylaxis. Studies demonstrate that pasturella infections typically manifest clinical signs and symptoms within 24 hours. Infections caused by other organisms typically develop within 72 hours [7, 38]. Therefore, patients who present greater than 72 hours from the initial bite with no signs of infection do not require antibiotic prophylaxis.

In summary, recent literature supports the use of prophylactic antibiotics in nontrivial human bites, mammalian bite wounds with high-risk characteristics, and/or mammalian bite wounds suffered by high-risk patients. There is no substitute for the value of adequate wound irrigation, cleansing, and debridement in the prevention of bite wound infections for all bites. If a bite wound meets the aforementioned criteria of high infection risk, it is important to consider the time since injury and the offending mammal in order to select the most appropriate antibiotic. These practices will help minimize mammalian bite wound infection rates, while preventing unnecessary side effects and risks of antibiotic prophylaxis.

Pitfall | Failure to provide appropriate wound after care instructions

There are several factors that affect the outcome of a wound. These include the choice of dressing placed on the wound and patient education regarding proper care of the wound. Experience demonstrates that there can be a wide variation in outcome despite proper wound preparation and suturing [39]. In order to optimize the cosmetic outcome of a wound, the physician must be mindful of the effects of UV light exposure and the choice of dressing applied to the wound.

> **KEY FACT** | Wounds exposed to sunlight within 6 months from the time of the injury can develop permanent hyperpigmentation.

The data to support avoidance of sun light exposure to a wound comes from plastic surgery and dermatology literature. In a retrospective study of patients undergoing dermabrasion, the authors observed that wounds exposed to sunlight within 6 months from the time of the injury can develop permanent hyperpigmentation [40]. Subsequent to this study, multiple animal experiments have demonstrated that UV light exposure on laser- and knife-induced wounds significantly alters normal skin structures and induces hyperpigmentation [41, 42]. Although these findings have not been investigated in humans, the recommendation is to use sunscreen products on a new wound for 6 months after epithelialization, which is typically complete within 48 hours. An optimal opportunity to discuss this with a patient is during a wound check visit. The patient should also be cautioned about the risk of hypersensitization to sunscreen products. It may be advantageous to recommend hypoallergenic products which are readily available over the counter.

The choice of dressing applied to a wound also impacts its cosmetic outcome. Dressings that provide moist, warm environments improve the rate of epithelialization [43]. Furthermore, they prevent contamination, sunlight exposure, and repeated trauma. Petroleum ointment and topical antibiotics such as bacitracin or triple antibiotic preparations provide the requisite moist environment for epithelialization. The value of antibiotic over petroleum ointment is controversial. In one prospective, randomized study topical antibiotics yielded lower infection rates [44]. However, a similar study published the following year found essentially no difference between antibiotic and petroleum ointments [45]. Some authors have suggested the use of antibiotic ointments, since there is no disadvantage linked to their use [1]. More recently, academic dermatology literature has warned against the routine use of bacitracin, citing that it is the seventh most common cause of contact dermatitis in North America. In addition to the adverse effects of contact dermatitis on cosmetic outcome, they cite more than 26 cases of anaphylaxis related to bacitracin use [46]. Of note, both topical antibiotics and petroleum products cause dissolving of cyanoacrylates and are not to be used on wounds closed with skin glue preparations.

Pearls for Improving Patient Outcomes

- When cleansing a wound, avoid antiseptic solutions or preparations, as they are tissue toxic. High-pressure irrigation with potable tap water is a safe and effective means of cleaning a wound.
- Clip or comb hair away from a wound rather than shaving at the skin.
- Wounds with high suspicion for retained foreign bodies should be further investigated with radiographs. If concern for radiolucent foreign bodies exists, CT or ultrasound is recommended.
- Bedside ultrasound is an efficient and cost-effective tool for localizing and assisting with the removal of foreign bodies.
- Maintain a high clinical suspicion for the presence of retained foreign bodies in plantar puncture wounds; especially if there is a delayed presentation.

- Universal prescription of prophylactic antibiotics for all bite wounds is not indicated. Clenched-fist human bite wounds are at highest risk for infection and mandate prophylactic antibiotic therapy.
- Optimal wound aftercare involves maintenance of a moist, warm environment until epithelialization occurs, followed by avoidance of UV light exposure for up to 6 months.

References

1. Wedmore IS. Wound care: modern evidence in the treatment of man's age-old injuries. *Emerg Med Pract* 2005; 7(3):1–24.
2. Pfaff JA, Moore GP. ED wound management: identifying and reducing risk. *ED Legal Lett* 2005; 16(9):97–108.
3. Singer AJ, Mach C, Thode HC, et al. Patient priorities with traumatic lacerations. *Am J Emerg Med* 2000; 18(6):683–86.
4. Howell JM, Chisholm CD. Outpatient wound preparation and care: a national survey. *Ann Emerg Med* 1992; 21(8):976–81.
5. Stevenson TR, Thacker JG, Rodeheaver GT, et al. Cleansing the traumatic wound by high pressure syringe irrigation. *JACEP* 1976; 5(1):17–21.
6. Longmire AW, Broom LA, Burch J. Wound infection following high-pressure syringe and needle irrigation. *Am J Emerg Med* 1987; 5(2):179–81.
7. Capellan O, Hollander JE. Management of lacerations in the emergency department. *Emerg Med Clin N Am* 2003; 21:205–31.
8. Hollander JE, Richman PB, Werblud M, et al. Irrigation in facial and scalp lacerations: does it alter outcome? *Ann Emerg Med* 1998; 31(1):73–77.
9. Oberg MS. Povidone–iodine solutions in traumatic wound preparations. *Am J Emerg Med* 1987; 5(6):553–55.
10. Oberg MS, Lindsey D. Do not put hydrogen peroxide or povidone–iodine into wounds. *Am J Dis Child* 1987; 141(1):27–28.
11. Dire DJ, Welsh AP. A comparison of wound irrigation solutions used in the emergency department. *Ann Emerg Med* 1990; 19(6):704–8.
12. Bansal BC, Wiebe RA, Perkins SD, et al. Tap water for irrigation of lacerations. *Am J Emerg Med* 2002; 20:469–72.
13. Valente JH, Forti RJ, Zandieh SO, et al. Wound irrigation in children: saline solution or tap water? *Ann Emerg Med* 2003; 41(5):609–16.
14. Tang K, Yeh JS, Sgouros S. The influence of hair shave on the infection rate in neurosurgery. Ped Neurosurg 2001; 35(1):13–7.
15. Horgan MA, Piatt JH. Shaving of the scalp may increase the rate of infection in CSF shunt surgery. *Ped Neurosurg* 1997; 26(4):180–4.
16. Seropian R, Reynolds BM. Wound infections after preoperative depilatory versus razor preparation. *Am J Surg* 1971; 121(3):251–4.
17. Perelman VS, Francis GJ, Rutledge T, et al. Sterile versus nonsterile gloves for repair of uncomplicated lacerations in the emergency department: a randomized controlled trial. *Ann Emerg Med* 2004; 43(3):362–70.
18. Singer AJ, Hollander JE (eds). Lacerations and acute wounds. Philadelphia: F.A. Davis Company, 2003.
19. Steele MT, Tran LV, Watson WA, et al. Retained glass foreign bodies in wounds: predictive value of wound characteristics, patient perception, and wound exploration. *Am J Emerg Med* 1998; 16(7):627–30.
20. Lammers RL, Magill T. Detection and management of foreign bodies in soft tissue. *Emerg Med Clin N Am* 1992; 10(4):767–81.
21. Schlager D. The use of ultrasound in the emergency department. Emerg *Med Clin N Am* 1997; 15(4):896–913.
22. Hung YT, Hung LK, Griffith JF, et al. Ultrasound for the detection of vegetative foreign body in hand – a case report. *Hand Surg* 2004; 9(1):83–87.
23. Graham DD. Ultrasound in the emergency department: detection of wooden foreign bodies in the soft tissues. *J Emerg Med* 2002; 22(1):75–79.
24. Dean AJ, Gronczewski CA, Constantino TG. Technique for emergency medicine bedside ultrasound identification of a radiolucent foreign body. *J Emerg Med* 2003; 24(3):303–08.
25. Dumarey A, De Maeseneer M, Ernst C. Large wooden foreign body in the hand: recognition of occult fragments with ultrasound. *Emerg Radiol* 2004; 10:337–39.
26. Schwab RA, Powers RD. Conservative therapy of plantar puncture wounds. *J Emerg Med* 1995; 13(3):291–5.
27. Fitzgerald RH, Cowan JDE. Puncture wounds of the foot. *Orthop Clin N Am* 1975; 6(4):965–72.
28. Weber EJ. Plantar puncture wounds: A survey to determine the incidence of infection. *J Accid & Emerg Med* 1996; 13(4):274–7.
29. Pennycook A, Makower R, O'Donnell AM. Puncture wounds of the foot: can infective complications be avoided? *J Roy Soc Med* 1994; 87(10):581–3.
30. Eidelman M, Bialik V, Miller Y, et al. Plantar puncture wounds in children: analysis of 80 hospitalized patients and late sequelae. *Isr Med Assoc J* 2003; 5(4):268–71.
31. Fisher MC, Goldsmith JF, Gilligan PH. Sneakers as a source of Pseudomonas aeruginosa in children with osteomyelitis following puncture wounds. *J Ped* 1985; 106(4):607–9.
32. Medeiros I, Saconato H. Antibiotic prophylaxis for mammalian bites. Cochrane Database of Systematic Reviews 2005; 4.
33. Dire DJ. Emergency management of dog and cat bite wounds. *Emerg Med Clin N Am* 1992; 10(4):719–36.
34. Taplitz RA. Managing bite wounds. *Postgrad Med* 2004; 116(2).
35. Smith MR, Walker A, Brenchley J. Barking up the wrong tree? A survey of dog bite wound management. *Emerg Med J* 2003; 20:253–55.
36. Broder J, Jerrard D, Olshaker J, et al. Low risk of infection in selected human bites treated without antibiotics. *Am J Emerg Med* 2004; 22(1):10–13.
37. Talan DA, Citron DM, Abrahamian FM, et al. Bacteriologic analysis of infected dog and cat bites. *New Engl J Med* 1999; 340(2):85–92.
38. Brook I. Management of human and animal bite wounds: an overview. *Adv Skin & Wound Care* 2005; 18(4):197–203.
39. Hollander JE, Blasko B, Singer AJ, et al. Poor correlation of short- and long-term appearance of repaired lacerations. *Acad Emerg Med* 1995; 2(11):983–7.
40. Ship AG, Weiss PR. Pigmentation after dermabrasion: an avoidable complication. *Plast Reconst Surg* 1985; 75(4):528–32.
41. Haedersal M, Bech-Thomsen N, Poulsen T, et al. Ultraviolet exposure influences laser-induced wounds, scars and hyperpigmentation: a murine study. *J Am Soc Plast Surg* 1998; 101(5):1315–22.
42. Davidson SF, Brantley SK, Das SK. The effects of ultraviolet radiation on wound healing. *Br J Plast Surg* 1991; 44(3):210–4.

43. Pollack SV. Wound healing: environmental factors affecting wound healing. *J Derm Surg Oncol* 1979; 5(6):477–81.

44. Dire DJ, Coppola M, Dwyer DA, et al. Prospective evaluation of topical antibiotics for preventing infections in uncomplicated soft-tissue wounds repaired in the ED. *Acad Emerg Med* 1995; 2(1):4–10.

45. Smack DP, Harrington AC, Dunn C, et al. Infection and allergy incidence in ambulatory surgery patients using white petrolatum vs. bacitracin ointment. A randomized controlled trial. *J Am Med Assoc* 1996; 276(12):972–7.

46. Jacob SE, James WD. Bacitracin after clean surgical procedures may be risky. *J Am Acad Derm* 2004; 51(6):1036.

Chapter 10 | **Management of the Pregnant Patient in the ED**

Kristine Thompson

Introduction

Caring for a pregnant patient can evoke anxiety in even the most seasoned emergency physicians (EP). The responsibility of ensuring the health of both the mother and fetus depends on accurate diagnosis and treatment of the mother without doing harm to the developing child. To make matters worse, pregnancy produces physiologic changes that lead to atypical presentations of illness and misinterpretation of diagnostic studies. This section includes some of the most common and most deadly pitfalls encountered in the care of a pregnant patient.

Pitfall | **Failure to suspect pregnancy**

> KEY FACT | **All women of childbearing age should be assumed to be pregnant until proven otherwise, regardless of sexual and menstrual history.**

While it seems obvious, the pearl here is to trust no one. All women of childbearing age should be presumed to be pregnant until proven otherwise. Every emergency department (ED) physician has a story of a patient who has a positive pregnancy test after being assured that there was "no chance" that she could be pregnant. In fact, one study found that 10% of women with abdominal pain or vaginal bleeding and a positive pregnancy test had denied the possibility of pregnancy [1]. Unless there is an operative report of a complete hysterectomy and bilateral oophrectomy, obtain a pregnancy test regardless of the sexual and menstrual history.

Pitfall | **Failure to detect ectopic due to heterotopic pregnancy**

> KEY FACT | **Visualization of an intrauterine pregnancy in patients with risk factors for heterotopic pregnancy does not exclude ectopic pregnancy.**

Heterotopic pregnancies are rare in the general population; however with the increasing incidence of pelvic inflammatory disease and in vitro fertilization (IVF), these cases are becoming more frequent with some estimates as high as 1:100 after assisted reproductive technology procedures [2].

Traditionally, ectopic pregnancy was ruled out once an intrauterine pregnancy (IUP) was identified. However, the increasing rate of IVF and resultant increase in heterotopic pregnancy necessitates a more careful interpretation of the ultrasound examination. The presence of a viable IUP does not rule out a heterotopic pregnancy unless the remainder of the exam is completely normal. Findings such as free fluid in the abdomen or abnormal appearing adnexae should be considered heterotopic pregnancy until proven otherwise, especially in patients who have conceived using assisted reproductive technology. Identification of an IUP in patients who have conceived using IVF who have signs and symptoms consistent with ectopic pregnancy should not be used to definitively rule out ectopic pregnancy. If unstable, these patients should be treated as if they have a rupturing ectopic pregnancy. If stable and close follow-up is available, they can be dismissed after consultation with their obstetrician.

Pitfall | **Failure to correctly interpret vital signs and lab values in the setting of pregnancy**

> KEY FACT | **Pregnancy physiology must be considered when interpreting vital signs and labs.**

The physiologic changes of pregnancy affect nearly all organ systems leading to changes in what are considered "normal" values for vital signs and many diagnostic studies. Misinterpretation of these indices can lead to missed diagnoses. Recall that values considered normal in the majority of the population can be a sign of significant pathology in the pregnant patient. A list of clinically significant changes is provided in Table 10.1. For a complete review, please refer to the maternal physiology section in the 22nd edition of Williams Obstetrics, 2005 [3].

Pitfall | **Failure to document Rh status and offer alloimmunization prophylaxis to patients at risk for maternal–fetal hemorrhage**

Screening for Rh status and offering anti-D immune globulin to pregnant patients who are at risk for maternal–fetal hemorrhage is critical in the ED. In order to be most effective,

Table 10.1 Normal physiological changes during pregnancy.

Blood pressure	Decreases 2nd trimester, then approaches baseline at term. Pathologic if >30 mmHg systolic or 15 mmHg diastolic over baseline, sustained >6 h
Heart rate	Increases 10–15 beats/min at rest
Respiratory rate	Unchanged, but hyperpnea is common, increased tidal volume, lower PCO_2, mild respiratory alkalosis is normal – hypoxemia occurs much more rapidly with hypoventilation or apnea
Hemoglobin	Lower – anemic if <11 g/dl in 1st and 3rd trimester, <10.5 in 2nd (CDC criteria for anemia in children and in childbearing-aged women. *MMWR* 1989; 38(22):400)
Plasma volume	Increases 50% (or 1500 ml) – significant blood loss may occur before clinical signs appear
Leukocyte count	Can be slightly higher, but depressed PMN function leading to "immunosuppressed state" (Krause P. Host defenses during pregnancy: Neutrophil chemotaxis and adherence. *Am J Obstet Gynecol* 1987; 157:274)
PT, PTT	Shortened secondary to increased levels of coagulation factors, plasma fibrinogen increases 50% – hypercoaguable state
Sedimentation rate	Increased
Serum Bicarbonate	Decreased (19–20 meq/l) – compensation for respiratory alkalosis
BUN, Creatinine,	Increased GFR, creatinine decreased (upper limit
GFR	of normal is 0.8 mg/dl)
Urinalysis	Small amount of glycosuria is normal, large may indicate gestational diabetes, proteinuria and hematuria are pathologic

prophylaxis must be given within 72 h of exposure. Although patients at risk are frequently seen in the ED, surveys have demonstrated that physicians fail to perform an Rh type and appropriately treat those who could benefit from immune globulin in approximately 85% of cases [4, 5]. The reasons that this intervention is so frequently missed are not clear but may include deferring the decision to the follow-up physician or lack of familiarity with the current guidelines. Failure to provide prophylaxis to an Rh negative mother who is exposed to Rh positive blood from her fetus will result in alloimmunization approximately 16% of the time [6]. The danger is the resulting insult to fetal red cells in subsequent pregnancies leading to varying degrees of fetal injury ranging from mild hemolytic anemia to fetal demise.

Controversy exists as to which patients have a high enough risk of exposure to warrant prophylaxis. The most current recommendations from the American College of Obstetricians and Gynecologists are summarized below [7].

> Indications for Rh screening and prophylaxis in the ED (7):
>
> - Level A recommendation
>   - After a first trimester pregnancy loss
> - Level C recommendations
>   - Threatened abortion
>   - Second or third trimester antenatal bleeding (placenta previa, abruption)
>   - Abdominal trauma

The main area of debate is whether to offer immune globulin to patients with threatened abortions under 12 weeks gestation. To date, there have been no definitive studies examining the incidence of fetomaternal transfusion in this group. The Royal College of Obstetricians and Gynecologists do not recommend anti-D immune globulin in women with a viable fetus before 12 weeks gestation who experience a brief episode of spotting [8], whereas the US guidelines recommend "strong consideration" for providing immune globulin to this group.

Rh isoimmunization is a potentially devastating event that can be prevented with appropriate screening and therapy. Treating physicians must carefully consider the possibility of maternal-fetal hemorrhage in every pregnant patient. Although controversy still exists regarding what constitutes a significant exposure, the treatment carries little risk of harm and withholding it could have devastating consequences. All Rh negative women who have the potential to be exposed to an Rh positive fetus should be offered anti-D immune globulin in the ED.

Pitfall | **Failure to perform a timely perimortem cesarean section**

Perimortem cesarean section has the potential to be life saving for both mother and child. It is also one of the most stressful situations an EP will ever face. It is one of those procedures that is practiced, simulated, and tested, but rarely performed. The procedure itself is dramatic and intimidating, and the window of opportunity to maximize survival is brief. The decision to proceed must be made quickly, but physicians often hesitate hoping someone with more experience will arrive. Unfortunately, that hesitation can be costly as the best outcomes are seen if the child is delivered within 5 min of the loss of spontaneous maternal circulation [9].

> KEY FACT | **When the uterine height is 24 cm or greater, the fetus should be assumed viable and, when indicated, a perimortem cesarean section should be performed.**

The decision to proceed with perimortem cesarean section must take into account both the benefits to the mother and to the fetus. In cases where the mother has sustained a lethal injury, the procedure is done to save the life of the child. However, maternal hemodynamic status is often improved when the fetus is extracted [10]. Indications for the procedure include loss of spontaneous maternal circulation and evidence of a viable fetus. As a history is rarely available, the assessment of fetal viability must rely solely on physical examination. At 20 weeks gestation, the fundus should be at the level of the umbilicus. After 20 weeks, the gestational age roughly correlates with the distance in centimeters from the pubic symphysis to the uterine fundus. If the fundal height is at least 24 cm at the time of maternal cardiopulmonary arrest, perimortem cesarean delivery is indicated.

> KEY FACT | **When performing a perimortem cesarian section, CPR should be continued, vasopressors should be avoided, and massive fluid resuscitation should be continued.**

During the procedure itself, CPR should continue to maximize placental blood flow. Massive fluid resuscitation is continued in lieu of pressors as placental vasoconstriction may compromise fetal outcome. Do not stop to prepare the abdomen as this only delays delivery. Begin the procedure as soon as possible, but no later than 4 min after loss of maternal pulse to ensure delivery by 5 min. A pre-assembled perimortem cesarean delivery kit can save time and frustration, however if there is no time for preparation, a large scalpel is all that is required. Perform a vertical midline incision from the epigastrium to the symphysis pubis following the linea nigra if present. Rapidly cut through all layers of the abdomen until the uterus is exposed. Next, open the uterus through a midline incision, thereby avoiding the uterine vessels which attach laterally. The safest practice is to start the incision at the fundus with a scalpel, then extend it with something more blunt such as large scissors. Once the first incision is made into the uterus, place your hand inside between the fetus and the uterine wall to prevent injury to the child as you finish the incision. Deliver the child head first if possible. Hold the child in a position lower than the mother, suction the mouth, and then clamp and cut the umbilical cord.

EPs must be prepared to act quickly and efficiently in order to offer both patients the best chance of survival. Because this skill is used infrequently and under very stressful circumstances, it is critical that EPs are very familiar with both the indications and the technique. Practicing the scenario under simulated conditions provides an excellent opportunity to practice both the cognitive decision to initiate the procedure, as well as the psychomotor skills for its performance. The recent advances in simulator technology provide a great opportunity for physicians to enhance their skills in the management of this high risk, low incidence procedure.

Table 10.2 Radiation exposure with common ED diagnostic procedures (values from multiple sources).

Study	Fetal Radiation Exposure (mrad)
Chest X-ray (shielding abdomen)	0.02–0.07
Extremity	1–2
Abdomen (2 view)	250
Pelvis	150–200
VQ scan	100–500
CT pulmonary angiogram	100–900
CT abdomen and pelvis	3000–5000

Pitfall | Avoiding necessary radiologic imaging for fear of harm to the fetus

A common myth circulating in both the medical and lay communities is that routine X-rays are harmful and will lead to fetal anomalies if performed on a pregnant patient. In fact, the risk to the fetus for most imaging studies is minimal, while the risk of a missed diagnosis to both the mother and the fetus may be substantial. There is no increased risk to the fetus of anomalies, growth restriction, or abortion with radiation exposure of less than 5000 mrad [11]. There may be a slightly higher incidence of childhood leukemia, but only if the fetus is exposed to more than 1000–2000 mrad in the first trimester [12]. As demonstrated in Table 10.2, most emergency evaluations fall far short of the amount of radiation associated with harm to the fetus.

To date, there have been no adverse fetal effects reported with ultrasonography or MRI thus these are the diagnostic modalities of choice in pregnant patients. Non-ionic oral and intravenous contrast agents are also felt to be safe. However, iodinated agents have been associated with neonatal hypothyroidism and should be avoided [12].

The decision to use radiologic imaging in a pregnant patient must take into account the risk to the fetus, the risk of harm to the mother, and the risk to the mother and fetus of missing a diagnosis because of a reluctance to use available imaging. Although the health of the fetus must be considered, appropriate diagnostic imaging should not be withheld from pregnant patients.

Pitfall | Attributing dyspnea in pregnancy to a gravid uterus

Dyspnea is a very common complaint during the third trimester of pregnancy. It is estimated that 75% of women in their third trimester complain of shortness of breath. The gravid uterus causes mass effect on the diaphragm limiting excursion, progesterone induces a mild respiratory alkalosis, and oxygen consumption is increased all leading to the sensation of dyspnea. However, the dyspnea of pregnancy tends to worsen gradually as the pregnancy progresses. A sudden onset or worsening of dyspnea should not be attributed to the gravid uterus alone. Potentially life-threatening causes of dyspnea in pregnancy include severe mitral valve stenosis (MS), peripartum cardiomyopathy (PPCM), and pulmonary embolus.

Cardiogenic dyspnea is an uncommon, but dangerous cause of shortness of breath in pregnancy. MS is the most common valvular lesion newly diagnosed in pregnancy [13]. The physiologic rise in heart rate and stroke volume may greatly increase the pressure gradient across the narrowed mitral valve leading to increased left atrial pressure resulting in congestive heart failure and atrial arrhythmias.

PPCM is defined as a dilated cardiomyopathy distinct from a pre-existing cardiomyopathy worsened by the stressors of pregnancy. The cause is unknown, but thought to be most likely immunologic, drug induced, nutritional, familial, or infectious [14]. The challenge in recognizing PPCM is that it is rare and the symptoms mimic those of normal third trimester pregnancies. Complaints such as pedal edema, dizziness, dyspnea, and fatigue are common in both normal late pregnancy and early congestive heart failure. There are no specific criteria to help identify these patients. Instead, the diagnosis relies on clinical signs of heart failure, the timing of symptoms occurring in the last month of pregnancy or the first 3 months postpartum, and echocardiographic evidence of left ventricular systolic dysfunction. Because PPCM carries a high mortality, patients with signs of heart failure or rapidly worsening dyspnea should be referred for echocardiography.

Pregnancy is an established risk factor for the development of venous thromboembolism. It is associated with marked elevation of several coagulation factors and increased production of fibrin leading to a hypercoaguable state. In addition, the gravid uterus compresses the lower venous system making the legs vulnerable to stasis and the formation of clot. The risk of venous thromboembolism is five times higher in pregnant women than in non-pregnant women of the same age [15]. Although the incidence of thrombotic events in pregnancy is relatively low, it is the leading cause of maternal death in developed countries [16].

> KEY FACT | In pregnant patients with suspected PE, CT angiography is the test of choice.

Clinicians should not hesitate to order the appropriate studies to make an accurate diagnosis for fear of harm to the fetus. The health of the fetus is dependant on the health of the mother and a missed pulmonary embolism (PE) could be life threatening for both patients. The diagnostic algorithm mirrors that of someone who is not pregnant. The use of D-dimer to risk-stratify patients with pregnancy cannot be recommended. The pre-test probability for PE in the parturient is, by definition moderate, owing to the hypercoaguable state of pregnancy. This negates the value of the test because it is ideally suited for patients at a low baseline pretest probability

for disease. Ultrasound of the lower extremities is helpful if positive, but again, an isolated negative exam in a moderate probability patient is not sufficient to rule out the diagnosis. If DVT without PE is suspected, serial non-invasive extremity exams are recommended [17]. Ventilation–perfusion scans had been the screening test of choice for PE in pregnancy. However, increasing evidence is supporting the use of helical chest computed tomography (CT). Although this practice has historically been discouraged, recent studies have demonstrated a lower risk of radiation to the fetus than with VQ scanning [18] and a higher sensitivity to detect disease. Additionally, CT provides information about structures in the chest in addition to the pulmonary vasculature.

Once the diagnosis of PE is made, the mother will likely require anticoagulation with heparin for the remainder of pregnancy as warfarin is contraindicated. She will also need to consider prophylaxis in subsequent pregnancies. Thrombolytics have been used in pregnancy, but the risk of placental abruption and fetal death due to these medications is unknown thus their use should be limited to life-threatening situations [19].

Pitfall | Over reliance on physical exam and laboratory data to diagnose appendicitis

The diagnosis of appendicitis in pregnancy can be very challenging. The typical symptoms including nausea, vomiting, and anorexia are present in normal pregnancies. Leukocytosis and elevated CRP are normal in pregnancy and thus are not helpful in ruling in or excluding the diagnosis. There also limitations in the physical exam. The expected findings of rigidity, guarding, and rebound tenderness signaling peritoneal irritation are frequently absent as gradual stretching of the abdomen leads to peritoneal desensitization [20]. Interestingly, the most commonly discussed change in the physical exam of pregnant patients with appendicitis may be a myth. It is widely believed and taught that the appendix migrates laterally and into the right upper quadrant with progression of pregnancy. This is based on a study using barium radiographs done in 1932 [21], however more recent clinical studies demonstrate that appendiceal pain, even in pregnancy, is most commonly located in the right lower quadrant [22]. Mourad et al. found that more than 80% of gravid patients with appendicitis reported pain in the typical location of the right lower quadrant. A subsequent study also did not support the displacement of the appendix by the gravid uterus [23]. The migration theory is likely a myth that continues to be perpetuated because it intuitively makes sense.

> KEY FACT | Pregnant patients with suspected appendicitis should have a confirmatory ultrasound performed prior to surgery.

A diagnosis of appendicitis in pregnancy should not be based on exam and laboratory findings alone. Appendectomy during pregnancy is associated with a fetal loss/miscarriage rate of 5.6%. This climbs to 10% if the appendix is perforated [24]. Because an unnecessary appendectomy could have devastating consequences for the pregnancy, radiologic imaging should be utilized to support the diagnosis prior to operative intervention. The diagnostic modality of choice is ultrasound which has been shown to be around 84% sensitive. If it is a technically difficult study or the results are inconclusive, helical CT scanning is recommended. CT in non-pregnant patients has been demonstrated to have a sensitivity of 98%, and a small case series in pregnant patients found CT to be 100% sensitive [25]. Although the dose of radiation to the fetus is substantial at approximately 3000 mrad, it does not reach the level of radiation believed to be harmful to the fetus (5000 mrad). As MRI becomes more widely available, it may replace ultrasound as diagnostic modality of choice as it combines little risk of harm to the fetus with excellent anatomic visualization [26].

The diagnosis of appendicitis is often made by clinical exam alone. This practice is not recommended in gravid patients as appendectomy in pregnancy carries a significant risk of miscarriage and fetal loss. That being said, delay in diagnosis has been associated with higher rates of perforation and fetal compromise. A rapid and accurate diagnosis will ensure the best outcome for the mother and child. Although current surgical practice still includes diagnostic laparotomy based on high clinical suspicion, every effort should be made to avoid unnecessary appendectomy during pregnancy.

Pitfall | Failure to monitor patients who have sustained minor blunt trauma in the third trimester

Trauma in pregnancy is not uncommon complicating at least 1 in 12 pregnancies [27]. Blunt trauma is more common than penetrating, with the most common mechanisms including motor vehicle accidents, assaults, and falls. Of these, car accidents occur most frequently accounting for nearly 60% of blunt trauma in pregnancy [28]. Many of these accidents are minor and significant injury is not suspected. Unfortunately, what may seem like minimal injury to the mother can cause life-threatening consequences in the child. Without appropriate monitoring, placental abruption and uterine rupture may be missed.

> KEY FACT | **Abdominal pain, tenderness, and vaginal bleeding may be absent with placental abruption.**

Placental abruption is the most common cause of fetal demise outside of maternal death in blunt trauma. The shearing forces experienced in blunt trauma can lead to separation of the rigid placenta from the elastic uterine wall. Approximately 2–4% of pregnant women experiencing minor traumatic insults will suffer a placental abruption [29]. Clinical signs and symptoms such as vaginal bleeding, uterine or abdominal tenderness, and abdominal pain are helpful, but are not always present and cannot be relied upon. Ultrasound has been proposed as an initial screening exam, however it has a sensitivity of less than 50% for placental abruption [30]. In contrast, uterine irritability has been strongly associated with abruption [31]. Cardiotocographic monitoring (CTM) has emerged as the standard of care for all patients in the third trimester who sustain blunt trauma regardless of the severity of the mechanism of injury.

> KEY FACT | **All patients in the third trimester of pregnancy with any degree of blunt abdominal trauma require CTM for a minimum of 4 hours.**

Ideally, an obstetrician or obstetrical nurse would be present to review CTM data. However, EPs should be able to recognize signs of fetal distress and uterine irritability. Fetal distress is manifested by fetal tachycardia, bradycardia, loss of beat to beat variability, or recurrent fetal heart rate decelerations. The definition of uterine irritability after trauma varies in the literature, but is most commonly referred to as more than one contraction every 10–15 min. CMT monitoring should be initiated as soon as possible in the ED and continued for a minimum of 4 h. Those with uterine irritability require admission for prolonged CMT monitoring. Any sign of fetal distress after 24 weeks gestation is an indication for emergent cesarean section. In cases of minor trauma, patients without evidence of fetal distress or uterine irritability during 4 h of monitoring may be safely discharged home.

Pearls for Improving Patient Outcomes

- Assume all women of childbearing age are pregnant until proven otherwise.
- Suspect heterotopic pregnancy in pregnant patients with abdominal pain and a viable IUP in the setting of fertility-promoting techniques, or with free fluid or abnormal adnexae on ultrasound.
- Carefully interpret diagnostic studies and vital signs in pregnant patients.
- Consider the potential for maternal-fetal hemorrhage in all pregnant patients presenting to the ED. Provide anti-D immune globulin to all women at risk for isoimmunization.
- Do not withhold appropriate diagnostic imaging from pregnant patients at any period of gestation.
- Recognize the indications for and be prepared to perform an emergent cesarian section on the hemodynamically unstable pregnant patient with potentially viable fetus.
- Patients with acute or significant progressive dyspnea in pregnancy should be investigated for causes other than the gravid uterus.

- Utilize all available data, including radiologic studies, to make an accurate diagnosis of acute appendicitis and avoid unnecessary appendectomy.
- Patients with viable gestations require at least 4 h of CTM monitoring after even minor trauma.

References

1. Ramoska E. Reliability of patient history in determining the possibility of pregnancy. *Ann Emerg Med* 1989; 18:48–50.
2. Habana A. Cornual heterotopic pregnancy: contemporary management options. *Am J Obstet Gynecol* 2000; 182:1264–70.
3. Cunninham et al. Maternal Physiology. Williams Obstetrics, 22nd edition, New York: McGraw-Hill, 2005; pp 121–50.
4. Grant J. Underutilization of Rh prophylaxis in the emergency department: a retrospective survey. *Ann Emerg Med* 1991; 21:181–3.
5. Weinberg L. Use of anti-D immunoglobulin in the treatment of threatened miscarriage in the accident and emergency department. *Emerg Med J* 2001; 18:444–7.
6. Bowman J. Controversies in Rh prophylaxis. *Am J obstet Gynecol* 1985; 151:289–94.
7. ACOG practice bulletin. Prevention of Rh D alloimmunization. Number 4, May 1999. Clinical management guidelines for obstetrician–gynecologists. American College of Obstetrics and Gynecology. *Int J Gynecol Obstetr* 1999; 66(1):63–70.
8. Royal College of Obstetricians and Gynaecologist. *Green top Guidelines. Anti-D immunoglobulin for Rh prophylaxis.* London: RCOG, 2002.
9. Katz VL. Perimortem cesarean delivery. *Obstet gynecol* 1986; 68:571–6.
10. Katz VL. Perimortem cesarean delivery: Were our assumptions correct? *Am J Obstet Gynecol* 2005; 192:1916–21.
11. Brent R. The effect of embryonic and fetal exposure to X-ray, microwaves, and ultrasound: counseling the pregnant and non-pregnant patient about these risks. *Semin Oncol* 1989; 16:347–68.
12. Guidelines for diagnostic imaging during pregnancy. ACOG Committee Opinion No. 299, American College of Obstetricians and Gynecologists. *Obstet Gynecol* 2004; 104:647–51.
13. Elkayam et al. Valvular heart disease in pregnancy part I: native valves. *J Am Coll Cardiol* 2005; 46(2):223–30.
14. Ro, A. Peripartum cardiomyopathy. *Cardiology in Review* 2006; 14(1):35–42.
15. National Institutes of Health Consensus Development Conference. Prevention of venous thrombosis and pulmonary embolism. *J Am Med Assoc* 1986; 256: 744–9.
16. Berg C. et al. Pregnancy-related mortality in the United States, 1991–1997. *Obstet Gynecol* 2003; 101(2):289–96.
17. Toglia M. Venous thromboembolism during pregnancy. *New Engl J Med* 1996; 335(2):108–14.
18. Winer-Muram H. Pulmonary embolism in pregnant patients: fetal radiation dose with helical CT. *Radiology* 2002; 224:487–92.
19. Patel RK. Thrombolysis in pregnancy. *Thromb Haemost* 2003; 90:1216–17.
20. Martin C. Physiologic changes in pregnancy: surgical implications. *Clin Obstet Gynecol* 1994; 37:241–55.
21. Baer J. Appendicitis in pregnancy with changes in the position and axis of the normal appendix in pregnancy. *J Am Med Assoc* 1932; 98:1359–64.
22. Mourad J. Appendicitis in pregnancy: New information that contradicts long-held clinical beliefs. *Am J Obstet Gynecol* 2000; 182:1027–9.
23. Hodjati H. Location of the appendix in the gravid patient: a re-evaluation of the established concept. *Int J Gynaecol Obstetr* 2003; 81(3):245–7.
24. Cohen-Kerem R. Pregnancy outcome following non-obstetric surgical intervention. *Am J Surg* 2005; 190(3):467–3.
25. Castro M. The use of helical computed tomography in pregnancy for the diagnosis of acute appendicitis. *Am J Obstet Gynecol* 2001; 184:954–7.
26. Birchard K. MRI of acute abdominal and pelvic pain in pregnant patients.. *Am J Roentgenology* 2005; 184(2):452–8.
27. Rosenfeld J. Abdominal trauma in pregnancy: When is fetal monitory necessary? *Postgrad Med* 1990; 88:89–91.
28. Shah A. Trauma in pregnancy. *Emerg med Clin N Am* 2003; 21:615–29.
29. Rothenberger D. Blunt maternal trauma: a review of 103 cases. *J Trauma* 1978; 18(3):173–9.
30. Dahmus M. Blunt abdominal trauma: are there any predictive factors for abruption placentae or maternal-fetal distress. *Am J Obstet Gynecol* 1993; 169(4):1054–9.
31. Pearlman M. A prospective controlled study of outcome after trauma during pregnancy. *Am J Obstet Gynecol* 1990; 162(6):1502–10.

Chapter 11 | **Pediatric Care in the ED**

Ghazala Sharieff

Introduction

The care of children in the emergency department (ED) can be quite challenging as the patient may be non-verbal, extremely anxious or present with a vague history. Several high-risk areas have been identified in pediatric emergency medicine. A recent retrospective study by Steve Selbst et al. discovered that the most common diagnoses involved in pediatric lawsuits in the US were meningitis, appendicitis, arm fracture, and testicular torsion [1]. Other areas of potential liability include medication errors, delayed diagnosis of intussusception and inappropriate evaluation of fever in children. This chapter will discuss some of the more common pitfalls in the acute care of children.

Pitfall | **Overdiagnosis of otitis media**

The American Academy of Pediatrics and the American Academy of Family Physicians formed a subcommittee on management of acute otitis media (OM). Their published practice guideline was designed to give recommendations for management of acute OM in children 2 months to 12 years of age (Table 11.1) [2]. In order to diagnose acute OM the following must be present.

Table 11.1 Diagnostic Criteria for OM [2].

In order to diagnose acute OM the following must be present:
Acute onset of symptoms
Signs of middle ear infection
(a) Bulging TM
(b) Limited or absent mobility of the TM – middle ear effusion is best confirmed by pneumatic otoscopy! (Pooled sensitivity of 94% and specificity of 80%.)
(c) Otorrhea
(d) Air-fluid level behind the TM
Signs of middle-ear inflammation
(a) Distinct erythema of the TM or
(b) Distinct otalgia that interferes with normal activity or sleep

> KEY FACT | **Antibiotics can be safely withheld for 48 hours in children older than 6 months of age without severe disease.**

In addition, the subcommittee recommended an option to withhold antibiotics for 48 h in children over 6 months of age who do not have severe infections or temperatures greater than 39°C. Children who have severe disease or infants <6 months of age with confirmed OM using insufflation, should be treated. High-dose amoxicillin (80–90 mg/kg) is still the first line drug of choice.

Pitfall | **Failure to differentiate a simple febrile seizure from other causes of seizures**

It is imperative that emergency providers know the definition and age range for simple and complex febrile seizures. These characteristics are listed in Table 11.2. As an example of a potentially devastating error that can occur by misclassifying a seizure as being a simple febrile one, a 12-year-old girl presented to an ED with the report of a fever and a generalized seizure that lasted 10 min. The Emergency Physician (EP) noted that the patient was back to her baseline mental status and no further workup was initiated. A diagnosis of a simple febrile seizure was made and the patient was discharged home. She returned later that day with status epilepticus. She is now neurologically impaired as a result of encephalitis.

Table 11.2 Characteristics of a simple febrile seizure.

To qualify as a simple febrile seizure, it must:
Be a generalized seizure
Last <15 min
Not recur within a 24-h period
Occur in a patient aged 6 months to 5 years
Occur in a patient with no evidence of meningitis on examination

> KEY FACT | **Though patients with simple febrile seizures require only an age-appropriate fever workup, patients with worrisome features should undergo lumbar puncture.**

Therefore, a complex febrile seizure occurs when there is a focal seizure, more than one seizure in a 24-h period, or duration of seizure activity exceeding 15 min. The workup of a simple febrile seizure vastly differs from that which should be performed in patients with complex febrile seizures. Trainer et al. [3] noted that patients with simple febrile seizures had no higher incidence of serious bacterial illness than patients with febrile illnesses alone. Therefore, the authors concluded that patients with simple febrile seizures need only undergo an age-appropriate fever evaluation. Routine electrolyte testing, CT scans and EEG's are not necessary. Warden et al. [4] in a review article concluded that routine lumbar punctures are not necessary in children <12 months of age with simple febrile seizures. However, a fever evaluation should be performed that is appropriate for the patient's age. A lumbar puncture should be strongly considered in patients <18 month of age who have: (1) a history of irritability, decreased feeding, or lethargy; (2) a prolonged postical period; (3) physical examination findings of meningitis such as a bulging fontanelle, photophobia, severe headache, Kernig or Brudzinski signs; (4) an abnormal appearance or mental status findings on initial observation following the postictal period; (5) any complex febrile seizure features; or (6) pretreatment with antibiotics. If these factors are not present and the child is well appearing a lumbar puncture can be deferred. In children over 18 months of age who have no signs of CNS infections, lumbar puncture can also be safely deferred.

Pitfall | Over-reliance on the peripheral white blood cell (WBC) count to determine whether a child needs to have a lumbar puncture

> KEY FACT | The peripheral WBC count should not be used to identify patients requiring a workup for meningitis or serious bacterial illness.

For years the peripheral blood count has been used as a marker for identifying patients with serious bacterial illness. According to published fever policies, patients who have a peripheral WBC count between 5 and 15,000 cells/mm^3 without a significant bandemia have a low risk of serious bacterial illness [5, 6]. However, this theory has been recently challenged. In a study by Bonsu et al. [7], the peripheral WBC count was found to be an unreliable marker in patients with subsequent meningitis. The authors examined the presenting WBC count in 22 patients who were subsequently found to have bacterial meningitis based on cerebrospinal fluid (CSF) analysis. The median value of the peripheral WBC count for patients with bacterial meningitis was 10,200 cells/mm^3 versus a median peripheral WBC count of 11,200 cells/mm^3 for infants without bacterial meningitis. Alarmingly, if a WBC count of 15 k was used as the sole criteria to identify patients requiring evaluation for meningitis, 73% of patients would have erroneously been missed. If the cutoff was raised to 20 k, 96% of patients with

meningitis would not have been identified. Using peripheral WBC counts of 5–15 k as low-risk criteria would have failed to identify 41% of cases of bacterial meningitis. The same authors evaluated the utility of the WBC count to identify children at risk for bacteremia and again found this test to be an inaccurate screening tool [8].

A lumbar puncture should be performed if the patient has clinical findings that are consistent with meningitis such as extreme irritability or lethargy, petechiae or purpura, bulging fontanelle, prolonged seizure activity, or any other abnormal physical examination findings. The reliance on the peripheral WBC count to guide the decision on whether or not to perform a lumbar puncture or to obtain blood cultures will only be misleading and grant a false sense of security in the patient's differential diagnosis.

Pitfall | Misdosing medications for children

Furthermore, medication dosing errors are also frequent. In a retrospective chart review of 1532 children treated at a pediatric tertiary care hospital, prescribing errors were found in 10.1% (154/1532) of the charts [9]. The following variables accounting for an increased incidence of errors:

1. Patients seen between 4 a.m. and 8 a.m.
2. Patients with severe disease.
3. Medication ordered by a trainee – higher incidence at the beginning of the academic year.
4. Patients seen on weekends.

The most common drugs involved in errors were: acetaminophen, antibiotics, asthma medications and antihistamines. There were two severe errors (drug error that could cause death or that was ordered was not administered) including one case in which a child with meningitis did not receive antibiotic. The take-home message is that when dosing medications for children, 47.5% of errors were ranked as significant – a drug error that could cause a non-life-threatening consequence or less effective treatment (e.g. 10-fold lower dose of amoxicillin for OM).

> KEY FACT | The weight of children should only be recorded in kilograms and dosage calculations and concentrations must be checked prior to administration.

A common cause of medication errors is the lack of standardization of the units in which children are weighed. Medication dosing is typically determined by the weight of the individual in kilograms. If a child's weight is mistakenly reported in pounds and dosing is based on this number, serious medication errors can occur. Alternatively, even if the weight is recognized as being in pounds, errors can arise by miscalculating when converting to kilograms. As an example, a 10-day-old male presented to the ED with complaints of poor feeding and vomiting. His weight was recorded as 6 pounds. The attending physician calculated the newborn as weighing 13 kg (instead of 2.7 kg!) and ordered a 280 ml bolus of normal saline rather than the recommended bolus of 54 ml. The patient began to develop respiratory distress and seemed to have a delayed capillary refill after the bolus was administered. The baby was given a repeat bolus of 280 ml of normal saline. The patient subsequently required intubation and transfer to a pediatric facility due to fluid overload. It is imperative that children be weighed in kilograms and this should start from the very first measurement. Requiring an additional step to convert from pounds to kilograms is inherently fraught with error. The take-home message is that when dosing medications for children, clinicians must check and recheck the dosing to not only ensure that their calculations are correct but that the dose administered is the dose ordered. This is particularly true in the setting of the high-risk variables listed above.

Pitfall | **Diagnosing colic in an infant without ruling out other causes of crying**

While colic is a common cause of persistent crying in infancy, other serious causes must be considered and excluded. The classic definition of colic follow a "rule of 3's" first described by Wessel [10]. A child with colic typically cries for 3 h/day, 3 days/week for at least 3 weeks and this excessive crying typically resolves by age 3 months. The physical examination will help to determine the cause of crying in approximately 41% of patients [11]. A systematic approach in imperative and the infant should be fully undressed and examined. Hair tourniquet syndrome can easily be missed and there have been many case reports of infants with hair tourniquets not only around the digits but also around the penis and clitoris. Corneal abrasions are also in the differential diagnosis and are readily diagnosed by flourescein examination. Intussusception also presents with crying and colicky abdominal pain and therefore a high index of suspicion should be maintained in patients who are described by the parents as "drawing up their legs" and then returning to normal baseline in between episodes. "IT CRIES" is a useful mnemonic that has been described to highlight common causes of unexplained crying in infants (Table 11.3) [12]. It is important that life-threatening and readily treatable causes of unexplained crying are identified and managed appropriately.

Pitfall | **Relying on the physical appearance of a newborn to determine the need for a full sepsis evaluation**

Neonates are at high risk for serious infection and are typically infected with virulent bacteria (such as group B streptococci, *E. coli*, and *Listeria monocytogenes*). Group B streptococci, is

Table 11.3 Causes of crying in infants.

I–Infections: otitis media, urinary tract infection, meningitis
T–Trauma: consider head CT, skeletal survey, focused radiographs
C–Cardiac: Congestive heart failure, supraventricular tachycardia
R–Rectal fissure, reaction to medications (immunizations), reflux
I–Intussusception
E–Eye: corneal abrasion or ocular foreign body
S–Surgical disease such as inguinal hernia, testicular torsion
S–Strangulation: hair/fiber tourniquet syndrome

associated with high rates of meningitis (39%), non-meningeal foci of infection (10%), and sepsis (7%) [13].

Several criteria have been tested in order to determine which infants are at risk for serious bacterial illness. Baskin et al. described the "Boston criteria" for febrile children ≥38.0°C between 1 and 3 months of age presenting to the ED [14]. Infants were discharged after an injection of intramuscular ceftriaxone (50 mg/kg) if the child was well appearing and had no ear, soft tissue, joint or bone infections on physical examination. These patients must have had CSF with <10 WBC/high-power field (hpf), microscopic urinalysis with <10 WBC/hpf or urine dipstick negative for leukocyte esterase, peripheral WBC count <20,000/mm^3, and a normal chest X-ray in patients in whom a chest X-ray was obtained.

Baker et al. developed the Philadelphia criteria to identify neonates who were at low risk for serious bacterial illness [15]. Patients who looked well (as defined by an Infant Observation Score of 10 or less) and had a peripheral WBC count <15,000/mm^3, a band-to-neutrophil ratio of <0.2, uric acid with fewer than 10 WBC/hpf and few or no bacterial on a spun urine specimen, CSF with fewer than 8 WBC/mm^3 and a negative Gram stain, negative chest X-ray (obtained on all patients), and stool negative for blood and few or no WBC on microscopy (sent on those patients with watery diarrhea) were considered to have a negative screen and were not treated with antibiotics. The neonates that were placed into the high-risk category had a higher incidence of bacterial disease (18.6%) but 4.6% of neonates classified as low risk had a serious bacterial infection. Kadish et al. found a similar rate of SBI in neonates that they categorized as low risk when they retrospectively applied both the Philadelphia criteria and the Boston criteria [16].

Another screening tool known as the "Rochester criteria" has been applied to infants ≤60-day old into high- and low-risk groups [17]. The children who met these criteria looked well, had been previously healthy, and had no evidence of skin, soft tissue, bone, joint, or ear infection. Additionally, they had normal peripheral WBC counts (5–15,000/mm^3), normal absolute band counts (≤1500/mm^3), ≤10 WBC/hpf of spun urine sediment, and for those patients with diarrhea, ≤5 WBC/hpf on stool smear. The low-risk group identified children who were unlikely to have serious bacterial infection, with a negative predictive value of 98.9%.

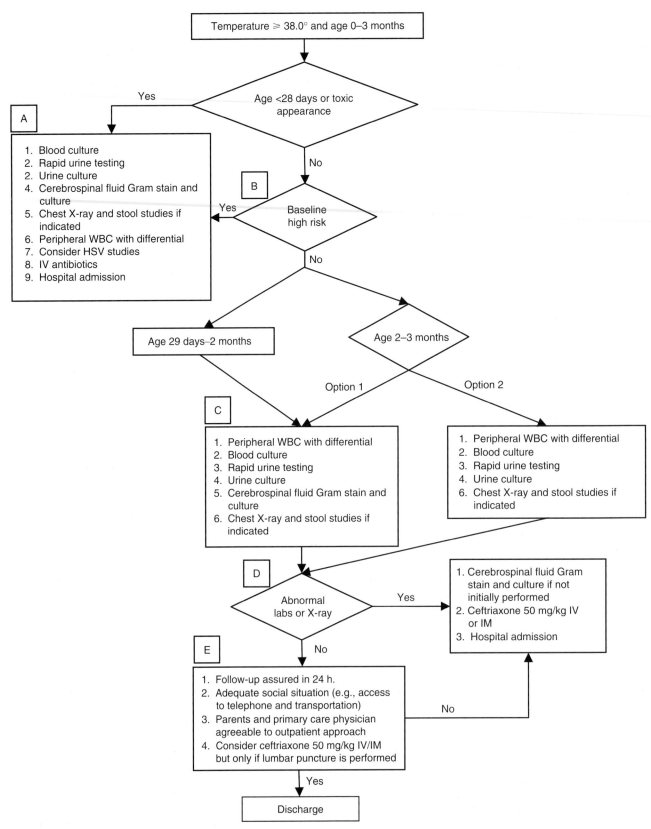

Figure 11.1 Guidelines for fever management in infants <3 months of age. Courtesy of Paul Ishimine. Children's Hospital and Health Center/University of California, San Diego. Fever without apparent source in children 0–3 months of age (adapted from [5, 6]).

Despite the number of different criteria available, none have been shown to be as accurate in the evaluation of the febrile neonate. Using the Rochester criteria, Jaskiewicz found that 2 of 227 children <30-day old who met low-risk criteria had serious bacterial illness (SBI) [18]. However, Ferrera et al. found a 6% incidence of serious bacterial illness in neonates that were retrospectively classified as low risk by the Rochester criteria [19]).

Another recent study compared the Philadelphia criteria to the Rochester criteria [20]. Infants <56 days of age who presented with fever were enrolled and all patients underwent a full sepsis evaluation (CBC, blood culture, urinalysis, urine culture and lumbar puncture). An investigator blinded to the final diagnosis assigned a risk category (low, intermediate or high risk of serious bacterial illness) based on the initial screening results. Ultimately the Rochester criteria would have failed to identify 2/65 infants with serious bacterial illness and the Philadelphia criteria would have missed one of these patients as well.

Because of inability to accurately predict serious infections in the <2-month-old age group, recommendations for these patients include obtaining blood cultures, urine for rapid urine testing, urine cultures, and lumbar puncture. Figures 11.1 and 11.2 show the current guidelines for fever evaluation in infants <3 months of age and infants and children 3–36 months of age [21].

Pitfall | **Misdiagnosing children with vomiting with "gastroenteritis"**

> KEY FACT | **Vomiting is a non-specific symptom and should not automatically be presumed to be caused by a self-limited infection. Serious infections, abdominal catastrophes, and inborn errors of metabolisms should be considered in all children presenting with this symptom.**

Vomiting is a non-specific symptom associated with many different disease processes. While rotavirus and other causes of gastroenteritis can present with vomiting as the initial complaint, in the absence of diarrhea, the clinician must maintain a high index of suspicion for serious pathology. Though one should always use extreme caution when making the diagnosis of "gastroenteritis" even greater caution should be exercised in children, especially those without diarrhea. It is also important to determine whether or not the emesis is bilious in nature. Bilious emesis is typically seen in patients with a bowel obstruction below the ampulla of Vater. Table 11.4 lists some causes of vomiting and the following case examples serve as a reminder to check for the underlying cause of vomiting in a child.

An 8-month-old female presents with vomiting and low-grade fever of 100.4°F. She looks dehydrated on examination but is not toxic appearing. Vitals signs show a heart rate of 160 beats/min, O_2 saturation of 100% and a respiratory rate of 20. The ED physician gives a bolus of IV fluids and since the patient is now tolerating fluids, she is discharged home. No laboratory data was obtained. The patient returned later that day with a heart rate of 180 beats/min, a temperature of 104°F, a systolic blood pressure of 60 mmHg and was minimally responsive on examination. She was found to have urosepsis. A common cause of vomiting is urinary tract infection and this is easy to check for. Bag urinalysis is not acceptable and has a high rate of contamination. Al-Orifi discovered that the contamination rate for bag urines was 68% versus 9% for catheterized specimens. A culture should also be sent, particularly in children <2 years of age as there is an approximate 10% incidence of bacteria without pyuria [22].

Another example of vomiting as a non-specific sign is that of a 1 year-old male who presented with non-bilious emesis and lethargy. Vital signs were within normal limits except for a heart rate of 170 beats/min. The patient seemed to have some mild abdominal discomfort but no focal tenderness. He did not have any diarrhea and was not febrile. The patient

Figure 11.1 (*Continued*)

A. Urine testing can be accomplished by either microscopy, Gram stain or urine dipstick. Chest X-rays are indicated in patients with hypoxia, tachypnea, abnormal lung sounds, or respiratory distress. Stool studies are indicated in patients with diarrhea. Herpes simplex virus testing should be considered in the presence of risk factors (see text for details). HSV testing is best accomplished by polymerase chain reaction or viral culture. Neonates should receive both ampicillin (50 mg/kg IV). Older children should receive ceftriaxone (50 mg/kg IV). A WBC count with differential may be sent but the results should not dissuade the clinician from pursuing a full evaluation and treatment with antibiotics.

B. Young patients who have increased underlying risk include children who were premature, had prolonged hospital stays after birth, those with underlying medical conditions, patients with indwelling medical devices, fever >5 days, or patients already on antibiotics.

C. Urine testing can be accomplished by either microscopy, Gram stain or urine dipstick. Chest X-rays are indicated in patients with hypoxia, tachypnea, abnormal lung sounds, or respiratory distress. Stool studies are indicated in patients with diarrhea.

D. Abnormal labs: Peripheral WBC count: <5000/mm³ or band-to-enutrophil ration: >0.2; Urine testing: 5 WBC/hpf, bacteria on Gram stain, or positive leukocyte esterase or nitrite; Cerebrospinal fluid: 8 WBC/mm³ or bacteria on Gram stain; Stool Specimen: 5 WBC/hpf; Chest X-ray: inflitrate on chest X-ray.

E. Administering ceftriaxone (50 mg/kg IV or IM) is optional, but should only be considered in patients who have undergone lumbar puncture. Patients who have not undergone lumbar puncture should not get ceftriaxone.

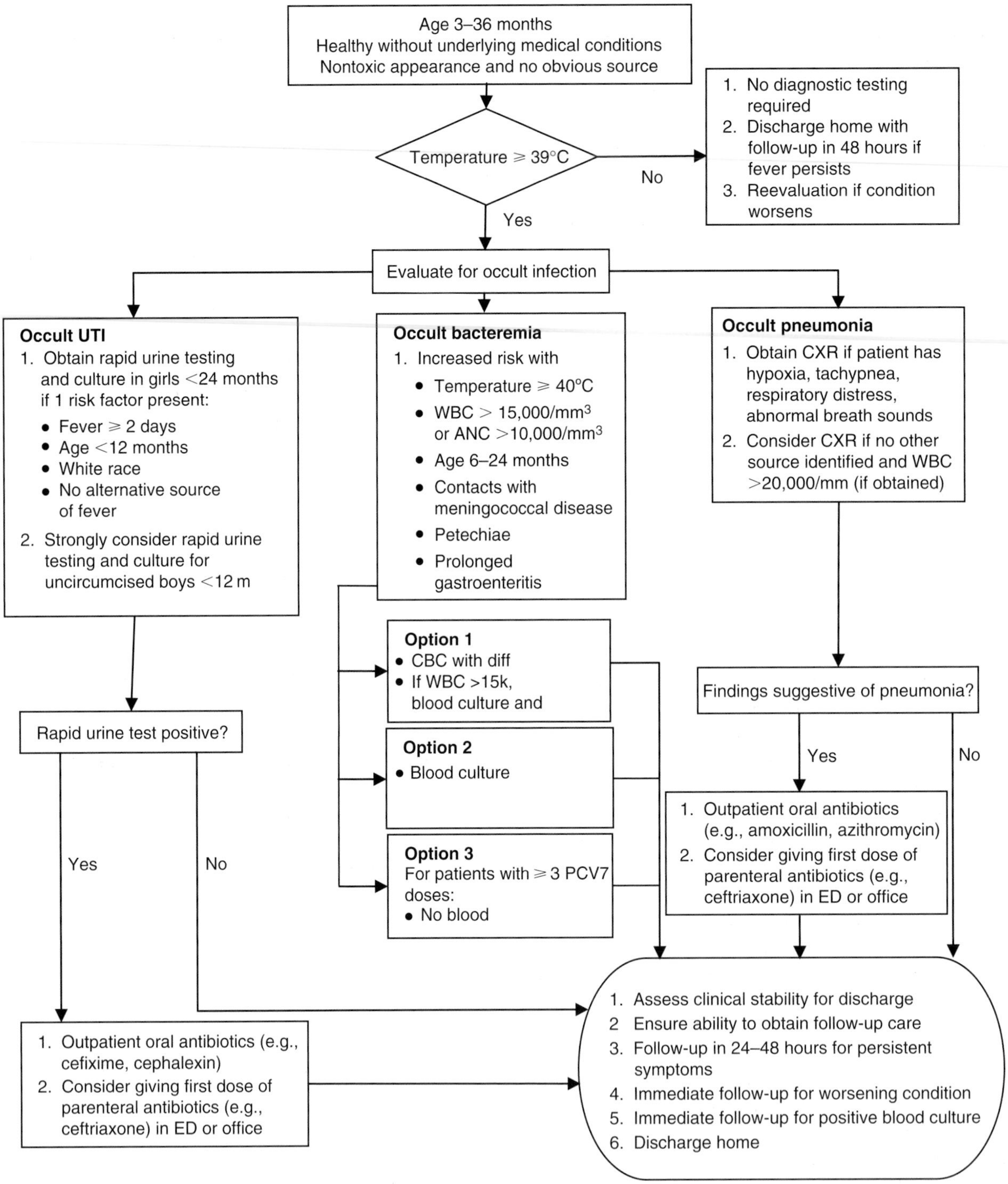

Figure 11.2 Guidelines for fever management in infants 3–36 months of age. Courtesy of Paul Ishimine, Children's Hospital and Health Center/University of California, San Diego (adapted from [5, 6]).

was given IV fluids and discharged home. He returned the next day with bilious emesis and frankly bloody stools. He underwent an unsuccessful barium enema and was taken to the operating room for a difficult reduction of an intussusception. The emergency care provider should have a high index of suspicion for this disease process in a child who present with vomiting only and either no fever or a low-grade fever. A rectal examination should be performed with the realization

that rectal bleeding is found in <40% of patients with proven intussusception. Furthermore, the classic triad of vomiting, paroxysmal pain and bloody stools is present in less than one third of patients [23]. However, the absence of bloody or heme-positive stools does not reliably rule out the presence of intussusception. If the history is suspicious, a kidneys, ureter, bladder (KUB) or preferably, a screening ultrasound can be performed. It is important to note that a normal plain radiograph

Table 11.4 Causes of vomiting in children.

Gastrointestinal/surgical	Infections	Other Causes
Appendicitis	Otitis media	Pregnancy
Cholecystitis	Meningitis	Drug ingestions
Cyclic vomiting	Pelvic inflammatory disease	Henoch Schonlein Purpura
Food poisoning	Respiratory disease → post-tussive emesis	Nephrolithiasis
Gastroesophageal reflux	(RSV, pertussis)	Uremia
Gastroenteritis	Streptococcal pharyngitis	*Metabolic*
Hepatitis	Urinary tract infection/pyelonephritis	Adrenal insufficiency
Hirschsprung disease		Diabetic ketoacidosis
Incarcerated hernia		Inborn errors of metabolism
Inflammatory bowel disease		*Neurologic*
Intussusception		Head trauma
Malrotation with midgut volvulus		Intracranial lesions/hemorrhage
Necrotizing enterocolitis		Migraine headache
Pancreatitis		Seizures
Peptic ulcer disease		Vertigo
Pyloric stenosis		
Small bowel obstruction		
Testicular torsion		

should not preclude further investigation. At our facility, we have had 2 patients within the last year who presented with classic histories for intussusception, vomiting and colicky abdominal pain, who had negative rectal examinations. The ED physican was astute enough to order enema studies in both of these children who did indeed have intussusception.

A final case for consideration is that of a 9-month-old female who presented to the ED with lethargy and vomiting. She did not have a fever. Her vital signs show a heart rate of 160 BPM, RR of 30, oxygen saturation of 99% and blood pressure of 90/50 mmHg. She appears to be encephalopathic on examination. CBC, CT scan and lumbar puncture are normal. Electrolytes are normal except for a glucose of 48 and a bicarbonate of 12 meq. An ammonia level was obtained at this point and was found to be markedly elevated. This child was ultimately diagnosed with an inborn error of metabolism. Key points to address in these patients are: (1) hydration status – most of these patients are dehydrated and many have been vomiting; (2) glucose replacement – these children are typically hypoglycemic and may require a central line to administer high dextrose infusions; and (3) these patients are at risk for infections as they may have low absolute neutrophil counts. In patients with organic acidemias, bicarbonate therapy (initial bolus of 1 meq/kg) may be life saving.

Pearls for Improving Patient Outcomes

- Utilize the published criteria to diagnose otitis media. In equivocal cases, withholding antibiotics for 48 h is safe to allow this entity to declare itself.

- Specific criteria should be used to differentiate simple from complex febrile seizures.
- Weigh children in kilograms not pounds.
- Do not rely on the peripheral WBC count to determine whether or not to perform a lumbar puncture on an infant.
- Do not diagnose colic without first searching for other causes of crying.
- Fully undress each child that you examine.
- Do not diagnose gastroenteritis in children who present with vomiting without diarrhea.

Acknowledgement

Special thanks to Paul Ishimine, MD for his tremendous help in preparing the fever section.

References

1. Selbst SM, Friedman MJ, Singh SB. Epidemiology and etiology of malpractice lawsuits involving children in US emergency departments and urgent care centers. *Pediatr Emerg Care* 2005; 21:165–9.
2. American Academy of Pediatrics and American Academy of Family Physicians. Subcommittee on management of acute otitis media. Diagnosis and Management of acute otitis media. *Pediatrics* 2004; 113:1451–65.
3. Trainor JL, Hampers LC, Krug SE, Listernick R. Children with first-time simple febrile seizures are at low risk of serious bacterial illness. *Acad Emerg Med* 2001; 8:781–7.

4. Warden CR, Zibulewsky J, Mace S, Gold C, Gausche-Hill M. Evaluation and management of febrile seizures in the out-of-hospital and emergency department settings. *Ann Emerg Med* 2003; 41:215–22.

5. American College of Emergency Physicians Clinical Policies Committee; American College of Emergency Physicians Clinical Policies Subcommittee on Pediatric Fever. Clinical policy for children younger than three years presenting to the emergency department with fever. *Ann Emerg Med* 2003; 42:530–45.

6. Baraff LJ. Management of fever without source in infants and children. *Ann Emerg Med* 2000 Dec; 36(6):602–14.

7. Bonsu B, Harper M. Utility of the peripheral blood white blood cell count for identifying sick young infants who need lumbar puncture. *Ann Emerg Med* 2003; 41:206–14.

8. Bonsu B, Harper M. Identifying febrile young infants with bacteremia: Is the peripheral white blood cell count an accurate screen? *Ann Emerg Med* 2003; 42(2):216–25.

9. Kizer E, Scolnik D, Macpherson A, et al. Variables associated with medication errors in pediatric emergency medicine. *Pediatrics* 2002; 110;737–42.

10. Wessel MA, Cobb JC, Jackson EB, et al. Paroxysmal fussing in infancy sometimes called colic. *Pediatrics* 1954; 14:421–34.

11. Poole SR. The infant with acute, unexplained, excessive crying. *Pediatrics* 1991; 88:450–5.

12. Herman M, Nelson R. Critical Decision in emergency medicine 2006; 20:2–10.

13. Pena BM, Harper MB, Fleisher GR. Occult bacteremia with group B streptococci in an outpatient setting. *Pediatrics* 1998; 102:67–72.

14. Baskin MN, O'Rourke EJ, Fleisher GR. Outpatient treatment of febrile infants 28 to 89 days of age with intramuscular administration of ceftriaxone. *J Pediatr* 1992; 120(1):22–7.

15. Baker MD, Bell LM, Avner JR. Outpatient management without antibiotics of fever in selected infants. *New Engl J Med* 1993; 329(20):1437–41.

16. Kadish HA, Loveridge B, Tobey J, Bolte RG, Corneli HM. Applying outpatient protocols in febrile infants 1–28 days of age: can the threshold be lowered? *Clin Pediatr* 2000; 39:81–8.

17. Dagan R, Sofer S, Phillip M, Shachak E. Ambulatory care of febrile infants younger than 2 months of age classified as being at low risk for having serious bacterial infections. *J Pediatr* 1988; 112(3):355–60.

18. Jaskiewicz JA, McCarthy CA, Richardson AC, et al. Febrile infants at low risk for serious bacterial infection – an appraisal of the Rochester criteria and implications for management. Febrile Infant Collaborative Study Group. *Pediatrics* 1994; 94(3):390–6.

19. Ferrera PC, Bartfield JM, Snyder HS. Neonatal fever: utility of the Rochester criteria in determining low risk for serious bacterial infections. *Am J Emerg Med* 1997; 15(3):299–302.

20. Garra G, Cunningham SJ, Crain EF. Reappraisal of criteria used to predict serious bacterial illness in febrile illness in febrile infants less than 8 weeks of age. *Acad Emerg Med* 2005; 12:921–5.

21. Ishimine P. Fever without source in children 0–36 months of age. *Pediatr Clin N Am* 2006; 53:167–94.

22. Al-Orifi F, McGillivray D, Tange S, et al. Urine culture from bag specimens in young children: are the risks too high? *J Pediatr* 2000; 137(2):221–6.

23. Yamamoto LG, Morita SY, Boychuk RB, et al. Stool appearance in intussusception: assessing the value of the term "currant jelly". *Am J Emerg Med* 1997; 15:293.

Chapter 12 | Management of Hematology/Oncology Patients in the ED

Robert L. Rogers

Introduction

The number of patients living with some form of hematologic or solid organ malignancy is rising. As treatment efficacy continues to improve, the number of patients with malignancies is increasing. Emergency physicians (EP) can expect to see increasing numbers of patients with these diseases presenting to emergency departments (EDs). Cancer is currently the second leading cause of death in the US, and it is estimated that one death in four is due to cancer [1].

Most of the oncologic urgencies and emergencies that present to EDs are actually, to some degree, amenable to therapy or intervention. Patients with these malignancies may present with a condition that, once treated, will allow them to lead relatively normal lives. Since hematologic and oncologic malignancies are so common, EPs must be experts in the recognition and initial management of cancer-related emergencies.

From a practical standpoint, hematologic and oncologic emergencies can be divided into three main categories: infectious, mechanical, and metabolic. The most important infectious complication is fever in the setting of neutropenia. Mechanical emergencies include airway obstruction, superior vena cava (SVC) syndrome, cardiac tamponade, and spinal cord compression. Metabolic emergencies make up the third group of emergencies and include entities such as the hyperviscosity syndrome, hypercalcemia, syndrome of inappropriate antidiuretic hormone secretion (SIADH), and acute tumor lysis syndrome. Because of some of the unique characteristics of cancer patients, it is essential that EPs seek out and treat these emergencies to optimize the outcomes for their patients.

The purpose of the following review is to emphasize the subtleties and atypical nature of some of the more common hematologic and oncologic urgencies and emergencies, and to highlight important diagnostic and treatment errors that occur in daily clinical practice. By having an appreciation of non-classic disease presentations and the clinical errors that occur in these patients, the EP can truly have an impact on morbidity and mortality in the cancer patient.

Pitfall | Failure to recognize and rapidly initiate appropriate antibiotic therapy when treating neutropenic fever

Of all the emergencies in hematology and oncology, fever in the setting of neutropenia is one for which expeditious recognition and management may significantly lessen morbidity and mortality. Rapid treatment of this condition is only possible if the treating physician recognizes that a pre-existing hematologic or oncologic diagnosis exists or that chemotherapy has been recently instituted. Absent of a hematologic malignancy treated by chemotherapy, other conditions that lead to neutropenia, such as agranulocytosis are quite rare.

> KEY FACT | **Afebrile patients who report a history of fever should be treated as if they are currently febrile.**

Neutropenia is said to exist when the total white blood cell (WBC) count is <500 cells/μl or a count of <1000 cells/μl with an anticipated decrease to <500 cells/μl. Most patients will have their nadir between 2 and 4 weeks after chemotherapy is initiated. Thus, patients currently receiving chemotherapy with a total WBC count <1000/μl may be on their way to approaching 500 cells/μl, depending on the time frame. In equivocal cases, the patient's oncologist should be contacted to collaboratively develop a treatment plan with the EP. Rates of serious infection climb significantly when total WBC counts fall below 500 cells/μl [2]. Fever in the neutropenic patient is present if the temperature exceeds >38.3° (101°F) or if the temperature = 38.0°C (100.4°F) for >1. Special care must be taken with patients who complain of fever but who arrive afebrile. Patients who report a fever meeting the above criteria prior to arrival in the ED should be treated as if they have a fever.

Patients with neutropenia may have few of the classic signs and symptoms of bacterial infections because of an inadequate number of circulating WBCs. Specific examples of altered presentations include the following:

1. A patient with a significant pneumonia may have no cough and no infiltrates on plain film.
2. A patient with a urinary tract infection may present in a subtle fashion because WBCs do not deposit in the urinary tract and produce the typical symptoms of dysuria and frequency.
3. Meningitis may present without clinical evidence of meningismus or cerebral spinal fluid pleocytosis.

Therefore, febrile patients with confirmed or suspected neutropenia should have cultures of blood and urine obtained and a chest X-ray performed. It is important to initiate empiric antibiotic therapy early and to provide broad coverage since the source of infection is often unknown. There is some data that a chest computed tomography (CT) may be the best initial choice to evaluate for pulmonary infection. Neutropenic patients with significant pulmonary infections, such as aspergillosis, may have a normal chest X-ray despite a remarkably abnormal chest CT [2]. If the patient has an indwelling central line in place, at least one set of blood cultures should be obtained through the line. Fever in the setting of neutropenia can rapidly deteriorate despite initially being stable. A thorough physical examination should always be performed to search for an underlying infection.

> KEY FACT | Appropriate initial empiric antibiotic choices include a third or fourth-generation cephalosporin a carbapenum. Vancomycin should be added for patients at risk for MRSA.

Progression of infection in neutropenic patients may be rapid, so empiric therapy should be started promptly at onset of fever. Initial antibiotic therapy should be tailored to the suspected offending pathogens. In the not too distant past, neutropenic patients were empirically treated with two antibiotics, typically a third-generation cephalosporin in combination with an aminoglycoside. Gram-negative bacilli, including Pseudomonas, *Escherichia coli*, and Klebsiella, have been the most common offending pathogens. Recently, however, there has been an increase in the rate of infections caused by gram-positive bacteria, many of them being methicillin-resistant organisms [2]. *Staphylococcus aureus* and coagulase-negative staphylococci are the most common causes, particularly if the patient has an indwelling catheter for chemotherapy or transfusion. There is now evidence to support single agent antimicrobial therapy. A third- or fourth-generation cephalosporin (ceftazidime or cefipime) or a carbapenem (imipenem–cilastatin or meropenem) can be used as monotherapy [2]. Including vancomycin in the treatment regimen would be indicated if a catheter-related infection is suspected, if the patient has known colonization with methicillin-resistant *Staphylococcus aureus* (MRSA), positive blood culture results with gram-positive bacteria before an identification is available, or if hypotension or sepsis is present [2].

Pitfall | Failure to identify malignant spinal cord compressive lesions

Back pain is a common and generally benign complaint encountered in the ED. As such, it is easy to minimize the etiology of patients with this complaint. In patients with a history of malignancy, spinal metastases must be considered. What can EPs do to lessen their risk of missing this potentially catastrophic entity? And what therapies can be rapidly instituted to lessen morbidity?

As many as 5% of all cancer patients will develop metastases to the spine and spinal cord at some point in the course of their disease [3]. Epidural spinal cord compression is a devastating complication of many malignancies, including breast, lung, and prostate cancer. Epidural spinal cord compression may be the first clinical manifestation of malignancy. Patient outcomes have been shown to be related to early diagnosis and rapid institution of therapy [4]. This may offer patients with advanced cancer the opportunity to maximize their quality of life during their final days.

Often, patients with a known diagnosis of cancer (breast, lung, prostate, renal) present for evaluation of back pain or new onset radiculopathy. EPs should maintain a high index of suspicion for potentially dangerous back pain entities, such as cancer, cauda equina syndrome, and abdominal aortic aneurysm, Any patient with a known history of cancer, no matter how remote, should be worked-up for this entity if the back pain is unexplained. Likewise, in patients with recent weight loss or other signs or symptoms of malignancy such as unexplained fever, an undiagnosed malignancy should be considered. There have been some case reports of recurrence of a previously diagnosed and treated cancer presenting as an epidural metastasis with or without cord compression [5].

> KEY FACT | Back pain that with neurological findings, atypical features, or in patients with symptoms suggestive of undiagnosed cancer should have urgent followup arranged.

Patients with early spinal cord compression may present with a variety of clinical findings. Common complaints include numbness, tingling, sensory loss, bowel or bladder incontinence, or abnormalities of proprioception, such as loss of vibratory sense. A detailed motor, sensory, and deep tendon reflex examination should be performed in all patients with suspected spinal cord compression, as well as observation of gait and evaluation of sphincter tone. Back pain worsened by particular maneuvers, such as coughing or lying in a supine position, should be considered suspect, as should pain that is worse at night. Most mechanical back pain entities do not cause worsening of pain with these maneuvers. New-onset radiculopathy from compression of a spinal root may also be the first manifestation of tumor. Many cases of spinal cord metastasis have been missed because of failure to consider metastasis to the epidural space and spine [5].

> KEY FACT | Patients with suspected spinal malignancies require magnetic resonance imaging (MRI) thought the urgency of the scan depends on the patients symptoms and findings. Patients with identified compressive lesions should receive corticosteroids and neurosurgical consultation.

For patients with suspected spinal lesions, MRI has become the modality of choice in most centers and should be obtained in all cases of suspected spinal cord compression. The timing of the study depends on the patients symptoms and findings. Patients with new motor deficits or symptoms consistent with cauda equina syndrome should have definitive imaging while in the ED. Those without findings should have urgent follow-up arranged so the study can be performed and followed-up rapidly. Patients with cord compression require neurosurgical consultation and high-dose corticosteroids.

Pitfall | **Failure to consider the diagnosis of SVC syndrome**

Generally, SVC syndrome is an urgency rather than an emergency. Two situations in which this entity becomes an emergency are cases in which cerebral edema or in which laryngeal edema have developed. This can lead to life-threatening cerebral herniation and airway compromise, respectively. In the past, the most common causes of SVC syndrome were tuberculosis, aortic aneurysm, and fibrosing mediastinitis. Today, lung carcinoma and other malignancies such as lymphoma are the most common causes. One particular cause with an increasing in prevalence is catheter-related SVC thrombosis [6].

Clinical manifestations of SVC syndrome are protean and depend on the degree of vena cava obstruction. Patients may be relatively asymptomatic and have only mild facial fullness when bending forward or may have florid symptoms of facial swelling, headache, and airway compromise. The key to understanding the variability of the clinical presentation is the anatomy of the azygous vein. The azygous vein is a large vessel that enters the proximal SCV and drains blood from the thorax. Obstruction above the level of the azygous entry point may lead to relatively few symptoms due to the ability of the azygous to decompress the upper extremities, head, and neck. If a compressive lesion or thrombus obstructs the SVC below the entry point there is no mechanism for upper torso, head, and neck decompression, and patients may present with marked venous collateral formation on the chest wall, neck, and shoulders and facial swelling on examination [7].

A clue to the diagnosis is the presence of asymmetric neck, chest, or upper arm venous distension. It is often helpful to compare the patient's appearance to that of a picture of the patient. If the patient does not have any photographs, a drivers license or other identification card picture can often be helpful to identify changes the patient's appearance.

Traditional teaching is that most patients will have a sensation of facial fullness, facial swelling, cough, variable arm swelling, and dilated neck and upper chest wall veins. SCV syndrome would not be a difficult diagnosis to make in this scenario. However, SNV syndrome may present with few if any clinical findings. The one symptom reported by many patients is a sensation of fullness when bending forward, or a vague, chronic cough. However, if venous decompression is able to occur, there will be no prominent veins or facial swelling. Thus, the diagnosis may not even be considered.

Treatment is aimed at relieving congestive symptoms. In cases where suspected or confirmed lung cancer or lymphoma is the cause, institution of radiation therapy may help lessen venous congestion and reduce upper torso, head, and neck venous pressure. Though SVC syndrome was previously considered an indication for emergent radiation therapy, this treatment should be reserved for patients with life-threatening laryngeal or cerebral edema. Patients with a confirmed or suspected diagnosis of SVC syndrome based on clinical grounds should undergo CT scanning to define the degree of SVC obstruction and to evaluate for the possibility of thrombotic SVC occlusion [8]. If there are no life-threatening features, this can be done as an outpatient if urgent follow-up can be arranged. Adjunctive treatments such as steroids and diuretic therapy may be used, particularly if head and neck edema is a prominent feature.

Pitfall | **Failure to identify malignant pericardial tamponade as a cause of dyspnea**

Pericardial effusions and tamponade are known complications of many malignancies including lung and breast cancer, lymphoma, and leukemia. Patients with malignancy may present for evaluation with a stable pericardial effusion, or may present in extremis or in cardiac arrest secondary to hemodynamically significant cardiac tamponade. Because malignancies are often identified late in their course, cardiac tamponade may be the initial manifestation of malignancy. In a small study of 23 cases of neoplastic cardiac tamponade, 8 cases were the initial presentation of the underlying malignancy [9].

> KEY FACT | **Patients with tamponade physiology are often hemodynamically stable on initial presentation.**

It is critical to remember that patients with tamponade physiology may be relatively hemodynamically stable [10]. Guberman et al. studied 56 cases of tamponade on a medical service and noted that most of the patients did not fit the classic description. Importantly, most of the patients had a normal blood pressure and no jugular venous distension on initial presentation [11]. Other studies have evaluated the classic physical examination findings and have found that as many as 30% of patients with tamponade lack classic findings [12]. More importantly, it is evident from the literature that patients with significant tamponade on the verge of decompensation and cardiac arrest may exhibit very few clinical indicators suggesting the severity of the tamponade [11]. Many cases of neoplastic cardiac tamponade present with dull or vague chest tightness, shortness of breath, and fatigue. Other clues to the diagnosis include low blood pressure, a narrowed pulse pressure, jugular venous distension, low voltage ECG, or cardiomegaly without evidence of heart failure on chest radiography, however their absence should not be used in isolation to exclude this process.

> KEY FACT | **Treatment of malignant pericardial effusion involves drainage of the pericardial fluid. The technique and timing must be determined by the hemodynamic stability of the patient.**

Treatment of neoplastic cardiac tamponade depends upon the hemodynamic stability of the patient. Unstable patients or patients who present in cardiac arrest (pulseless electrical activity) should undergo needle pericardiocentesis. In a cardiac arrest situation this is commonly performed blindly. For patients who are hemodyamically stable pericardiocentesis can also be performed by ECG guidance or under fluoroscopy. With the increased use of bedside ultrasonography in EDs, pericardial effusions can be more effectively localized and safely performed [13]. Consultation with a cardiologist and a cardiothoracic surgeon should be undertaken because in some cases a definitive procedure such as a pericardial drain or window will need to be performed.

Pitfall | **Failure to identify hyperviscosity syndrome as a cause for dyspnea or altered mental status**

Hyperviscosity syndrome and leukostasis syndrome may be one of the most difficult hematologic emergencies to detect in the ED. Hyperviscosity syndrome is caused by increased blood viscosity while leukostasis syndrome is caused by marked leukocytosis.

> KEY FACT | **Hyperviscosity syndrome must be considered in patients with mental status changes or dyspnea and a history of hematologic malignancy.**

Signs and symptoms of hyperviscosity typically manifest when serum viscosity reaches five times the viscosity of water. Normal human serum is 1.4 to 1.8 times as viscous as water. Clinical manifestations are directly related to high viscosity and can be caused by multiple hematologic disorders, such as Waldenstrom's macroglobulinemia, multiple myeloma, acute leukemia with blast crisis, and polycythemia vera [14]. Patients with a known diagnosis of any one of these disorders who present with mental status changes, unexplained dyspnea, or headache should be suspected of having a hyperviscosity syndrome and should have appropriate therapy instituted. Clinical presentations will be dictated by flow characteristics of different blood vessels and are directly

related to microcirculatory occlusion [15]. This may manifest as derangements in central nervous system (CNS) function or hypoxemia and respiratory failure.

The important dilemma for EPs is in detecting this disorder de novo in a patient without a known hematologic diagnosis. One clinical pearl is to consider a hyperviscous state in patients when the laboratory has trouble running their blood through the laboratory equipment. Serum viscosity is reported in Centipoises. A normal serum viscosity is less than 1.8, and clinical symptoms are rare unless serum viscosity is greater than 4.0 Centipoises. In some hospitals the test can be performed in an hour, whereas in others it is a send out laboratory test with a longer turnaround time. The EP should also strongly consider this diagnosis in cases of unexplained coma or unexplained shortness of breath [14]. Given that there is no known gold standard for diagnosis, EPs should have a high index of suspicion for this disorder in patients with clinical deterioration with an underlying hematologic disease.

Treatment in the ED should be aimed at lowering serum viscosity. If a patient already has a diagnosis, this will almost always involve consultation with the patient's hematologist. Therapy is instituted to correct the causative factor of the hyperviscosity syndrome. Management of this condition should involve lowering of the cellular or protein components of blood [15]. In cases of multiple myeloma, this might involve plasmapheresis to lower serum protein levels. The primary role of the EP is to assess the patient's airway, breathing, and circulation, initiate resuscitative efforts, and to begin aggressive intravenous hydration. Phlebotomy of 2–3 units of blood is also an effective temporizing treatment modality.

> KEY FACT | **Leukostasis syndrome is most commonly symptomatic when leukocyte counts approach 100,000/μl but can be seen with counts of 25000–50,000/μl**

Leukostasis, or hyperleukocytosis, is a condition defined by tissue hypoperfusion secondary to elevated WBCs. This is seen in some cases of acute leukemia. This particular syndrome is typically seen when total WBC counts approach 100,000/μl but can be seen in certain types of monoblastic leukemias when the total WBC count is only 25–50,000/μl [16].

As with hyperviscosity syndrome, the central nervous and pulmonary systems are the most commonly involved in leukostasis syndrome. Patients may present with new onset or unexplained shortness or breath, respiratory failure, and depressed mental status. Infiltration of the gastrointestinal (GI) tract or liver may lead to GI bleeding or liver failure [16]. Diagnosis is typically made in the setting of organ dysfunction and a markedly elevated peripheral WBC count.

> KEY FACT | **Patients with leukostasis syndrome should receive aggressive hydration and undergo whole blood phlebotomomy in the ED.**

Treatment requires a multifaceted approach. Aggressive intravenous hydration should be rapidly instituted in the ED. A hematologist should be contacted in order to plan definitive chemotherapy. In the ED, the key principles of treatment include measures to rapidly lower peripheral WBC counts and to prepare for the inevitable development of the tumor lysis syndrome. This syndrome is composed of hyperkalemia, hyperuricemia, hyperphosphatemia, and renal failure and results when leukemic blasts or lymphoma cells undergo cell death with release of intracellular contents [17, 18]. Treatments include oral administration of phosphate binders and allopurinol along with aggressive intravenous hydration [19]. An initial dose of 600 mg of oral allopurinol can be given in the ED. Alternatively, intravenous Rasbiricase, a recombinant urate oxidase, can be given in an initial dose of 0.05–0.2 mg/kg intravenously. This drug has been shown to be extremely effective at reducing serum urate levels and can prevent the development of acute renal failure [19]. The most commonly used phosphate binder is aluminum hydroxide and is generally given in a dose of 50–150 mg/kg orally daily. Leukapheresis or whole blood phlebotomy can be used to lower the white count until chemotherapy has begun. This can be performed in the ED as a temporizing measure until definitive care is undertaken. Whole blood phlebotomy can be performed by withdrawing 1–2 units of whole blood in an effort to temporarily lower serum viscosity. In addition, hydroxyurea in a dosage of 50–100 mg/kg daily can be given while awaiting chemotherapy.

KEY FACT | **Blood transfusion should be avoided in patients with leukostasis syndrome as it can worsen small vessel ischemia.**

Another important pitfall is transfusing red blood cells to these patients. The combination of WBCs, red blood cells, platelets, and other serum constituents make up an individual patient's *cytocrit*. The cytocrit is related to the serum viscosity. Higher the cytocrit, higher is the viscosity. Since many, if not most, patients with leukostasis have leukemia as the underlying diagnosis, almost all will be severely anemic secondary to bone marrow suppression. The temptation is to transfuse blood products. This should be performed with extreme caution since even small elevations of the patient's cytocrit may cause worsening small vessel ischemia and result in worsening hypoxia and CNS hemorrhage.

Pitfall | **Not Considering the Diagnosis of the SIADH and Failure to Appropriately Treat**

One of the more common oncologic entities seen in EDs is the SIADH. This syndrome is caused by release of antidiuretic hormone from ectopic sites such as a lung cancer or CNS infection and leads to hyponatremia. When severe, hyponatremia constitutes a true oncologic emergency [20].

Hyponatremia is the most frequent electrolyte disorder in clinical medicine. This frequently chronic and often stable condition may become life threatening when serum sodium concentration continues to fall and patients develop CNS manifestations such as coma or seizures. Symptoms may also include anorexia, weakness, confusion, and changes in mental status.

It is imperative that EPs know how fast to treat hyponatremia. The most feared complication of excessively rapid correction of hyponatremia is the osmotic demyelination syndrome (ODS), formerly known as central pontine myelinolysis (CPM), a devastating condition in which there is destruction of neurons and edema of the pons and midbrain [21]. It is generally agreed that acute, symptomatic hyponatremia (seizures or coma) should be treated aggressively to raise the serum sodium rapidly to a level above a theoretical seizure threshold. The literature most often quotes a level of somewhere between 120 and 130 meq/dl [21]. A good rule of thumb for dealing with hyponatremia in the ED is to correct chronic hyponatremia slowly and acute hyponatremia quickly. The problem with this traditional teaching is that most of the time EPs are presented with an ill-appearing hyponatremic patient with an unknown history and unknown duration of hyponatremia. Frequently the decision to institute therapy must be done with little if any past medical history.

KEY FACT | **Rapidity of correction of hyponatremia is determined by the patient's symptoms. Hypertonic saline should be reserved for those actively seizing. Normal saline or fluid restriction should be administered to those with milder disease.**

What is evident from the literature is that acute, symptomatic hyponatremia (seizures and/or coma) should be treated rapidly with hypertonic (3%) saline [21]. Hypertonic saline can be administered at a rate of approximately 1–2 cc/kg/h in order to raise the serum sodium by 2.5 meq/h. In the ED, this can be safely accomplished by administering 100–200 cc of 3% saline over a few hours. Thus, if a patient with a sodium of 105 is actively seizing, hypertonic saline is given to correct the serum level to the seizure threshold, somewhere around 115–120 meq/l. The whole point of this treatment is to raise the serum sodium by approximately 10 meq/l, which in many cases will stop seizure activity. The hypertonic saline should then be stopped. Frequent laboratory assessments must be performed to assure that the desired rate and level correction is not exceeded. It can also be determined precisely how much hypertonic saline to administer and how fast according to the patient's sodium level on presentation and the goal sodium level. Since this can be tedious and time consuming for the practicing EP, it is not discussed here. As a rule of thumb, hyponatremia that is chronic in nature should be corrected slowly at a rate of no more than 0.5 meq/h or 12 meq over a 24-h period. Treatment of mild hyponatremia secondary to SIADH includes free water restriction (500 cc – 1 l/day) with close follow-up by the patient's oncologist or administration of demeclocycline, a tetracycline derivative, which produces nephrogenic diabetes insipidus. It is usually given in a dose of 250 mg four times a day and is usually started after discussion with the patient's oncologist.

Pearls for Improving Patient Outcomes

- All febrile patients with a history of cancer undergoing treatment with chemotherapy should be considered to be neutropenic until proven otherwise. They should receive broad spectrum antibiotics early.
- Spinal metastasis and cord compression may be the first symptom of a malignancy.
- Neoplastic cardiac tamponade may be the first clinical manifestation of cancer. Cancer patients who present with unexplained cardiopulmonary symptoms should have this diagnosis ruled out.
- The diagnosis of hyperviscosity syndrome should be considered in all patients with hematologic malignancies who present with a constellation of unexplained signs and symptoms. Prompt institution of measures to decrease serum viscosity should be initiated in the ED.
- Blood transfusion is to be avoided unless absolutely necessary in patients with leukostasis syndrome.
- Hypertonic saline should be reserved for hyponatremic patients who are actively seizing or have altered mental status.

References

1. Current Clinical Issues-Cancer chemotherapy: Teaching old drugs new tricks. *Annals of Int Med* 2001; 135:1107–10.
2. Hughes WT, Armstrong D, Bodey GP, et al. Guidelines for the use of antimicrobial agents in neutropenic patients with cancer-IDSA guidelines. *Clin Infect Dis* 2002; 34:730–51.
3. Posner JB. Back pain and epidural spinal cord compression. *Med Clin N Am* 1987; 71:185–204.
4. Kim RY, Spencer SA, Meridith RF, et al. Extradural spinal cord compression: analysis of factors determining functional progress, prospective study. *Radiology* 1990; 176:279–82.
5. Helweg-Larson S, Sorensen PS. Symptoms and signs in metastatic spinal cord compression: a study of progression from first symptoms until diagnosis in 153 patients. *Eur J Cancer* 1994; 3A:396–99.
6. Nieto AF, Doty DB. Superior vena cava obstruction: clinical syndrome, etiology, and treatment. *Curr Probl Cancer* 1986; 10:441–84.
7. Maguire WM. Mechanical complications of cancer. *Emerg Med Clin N Am* 1993; 11:421–30.
8. Schwartz EE, Goodman LR, Haskin ME. Role of CT scanning in the superior vena cava syndrome. *Am J Clin Oncol* 1986; 9:71–78.
9. Haskel RJ, French WJ. Cardiac tamponade as the initial presentation of malignancy. *Chest* 1985; 88(1):70–73.
10. Kralstein J, Fishman WH. Malignant pericardial disease: diagnosis and treatment. *Cardiol Clin* 1987; 5:583–89.
11. Guberman BA, Fowler NO, Gueron M, et al. Cardiac tamponade in medical patients. *Circulation* 1981; 64(3):633–40.
12. Levine MJ, Lorell BH, Diver DJ, et al. Implications of echocardiographically-assisted diagnosis of pericardial tamponade in contemporary medical patients: detection before hemodynamic embarrassment. *J Am Coll Cardiol* 1991; 17(1): 59–65.
13. Blavais M. Incidence of pericardial effusion in patients presenting to the emergency department with unexplained dyspnea. *Acad Emerg Med* 2001; 8(12):1143–6.
14. Kwaan HC, Bongu A. The hyperviscosity syndromes. *Semin Thromb Hemost* 1999; 25(2):199–208.
15. Coppell J. Consider 'hyperviscosity syndrome' in unexplained breathlessness. *Acta Haematol* 2000; 104(1):52–53.
16. Markman M. Common complications and emergencies associated with cancer and its therapy. *Cleve Clin J Med* 1994; 12:105–14.
17. Arrambide K, Toto RD. Tumor lysis syndrome. *Semin Nephrol* 1993; 13:273–80.
18. Alkhuja S, Ulrich H. Acute renal failure from spontaneous acute tumor lysis syndrome: a case report and review of the literature. *Ren Fail* 2002; 24(2):227–32.
19. Davidson MB, Thakkar S, Hix JK, et al. Pathophysiology, clinical consequences, and treatment of tumor lysis syndrome. *Am J Med* 2004; 116:546–54.
20. Lin M, Liu SJ, Lim IT. Disorders of water imbalance. *Emerg Med Clin N Am* 2005; 23(3):749–70.
21. Adrogue HJ, Madias NE. Primary Care: Hyponatremia. *New Eng J Med* 2000; 342:1581–89.

Chapter 13 | Management of Intoxicated/Violent Patients

Yesha Patel & Gus M. Garmel

Introduction

Patients who are intoxicated, violent, or both often receive superficial or delayed medical evaluations in the emergency department (ED). A number of reasons for this exist, as these patients may be unpleasant, disrespectful to staff, and often have poor hygiene. Some staff may prefer that these patients be "quickly dispositioned," as they may not be comfortable caring for them, may not feel appreciated by them, or may feel their safety is threatened. Furthermore, these patients can be disruptive to the ED and other patients. Often, intoxicated or violent patients are given premature diagnoses based on stereotypes or presumptions, especially if they have had prior ED visits. They may be kept in the waiting room or relegated to corners of the department so that priority can be given to other patients.

Unfortunately, the management of intoxicated and violent patients involves several high-risk medical and legal issues. Both groups may have serious underlying illnesses that must be rapidly identified and addressed. At the same time, emergency physicians (EPs) need to institute appropriate measures to protect themselves, other staff, the patient, and innocent third parties. Finally, EPs must be aware of and comply with local, state, and federal regulations with respect to intoxicated and/or violent patients.

Pitfall | Failure to perform a comprehensive medical evaluation

> KEY FACT | **Ethanol has little or no odor. Correlation does not exist between the strength of odor on a patient's breath and his or her level of intoxication.**

Intoxicated patients should be evaluated with the assumption that an underlying medical or traumatic condition exists until proven otherwise. Some patients may appear intoxicated despite an alternative diagnosis causing their symptoms. Behaviors associated with intoxication, such as slurred speech, ataxia, sleepiness, or confusion may also be the result of metabolic disorders (hypoglycemia, hypoxia, uremia, Wernicke's encephalopathy, diabetic ketoacidosis, or electrolyte imbalances), neurological illnesses (trauma, ischemia, neoplasms, dementia, or postictal states), infections, or endocrinopathies. One reason clinicians may be misled is their over-reliance on a patient's breath odor. Ethanol has little or no odor. The odor that physicians misidentify comes from aromatic substances in an alcoholic drink, which persist even after the ethanol has been metabolized. Correlation does not exist between the strength of odor on a patient's breath and his or her level of intoxication.

Even if a patient is intoxicated, it remains imperative to consider and rule out co-existing illnesses and trauma. Some patients become intoxicated to mask the pain of underlying life-threatening conditions. Doing so alters the presentations typical of these conditions, leading to delayed or missed diagnoses. Patients who drink alcohol chronically are especially at increased risk for serious medical problems because of underlying liver disease, cardiomyopathies, and nutritional deficiencies. Furthermore, intoxicated patients are more likely to fall, experience closed head injuries, and have sequelae related to bleeding diatheses.

Violent patients also run the risk of having underlying medical illnesses missed, as their behavior is often attributed to underlying psychiatric diagnoses. One study reported that EPs documented "medically clear" in 80% of patients later identified to have medical disease [1]. Another study demonstrated that 46% of consecutive newly hospitalized psychiatric patients had an unrecognized medical illness that either caused or exacerbated their psychiatric illness [2]. While several psychiatric illnesses may cause violent behavior, organic (medical) illnesses are more commonly responsible. One frequently cited study of 100 consecutive alert adult ED patients with new psychiatric symptoms reported that 63 had an organic etiology for their symptoms [3].

Alcohol or drug intoxication and withdrawal are among the most common causes for violent behavior. Medication overdoses and drug–drug interactions are also commonly responsible. Elderly patients and patients taking psychiatric medications are at particular risk for drug toxicity due to polypharmacy, complicated dosing regimens, and narrow therapeutic windows. Metabolic, neurologic, infectious, and endocrine disorders must also be considered as underlying causes of violent behavior.

> KEY FACT | **Psychiatric conditions rarely present suddenly or with visual, tactile, or olfactory hallucinations.**

Missing an organic condition increases the morbidity of a patient who has been declared "medically clear" and admitted to a psychiatric ward, as further medical evaluation may be limited or not occur. Given the prevalence of missed medical diagnoses, it is wise to assume that patients exhibiting violent behavior have an associated organic illness until proven otherwise. Several screening criteria exist which may rapidly differentiate between medical and psychiatric etiologies (see Table 13.1). Disorientation, fluctuating levels of consciousness, abnormal vital signs, and age greater than 40 without previous psychiatric history strongly suggest organic illness [4]. In addition, psychiatric conditions rarely present suddenly or with visual, tactile, or olfactory hallucinations [5].

Table 13.1 Factors favoring organic illness over psychiatric illness.*

Age >40 or <12, without previous history of psychiatric illness
Abnormal vital signs
Abrupt onset of symptoms
Absent family history of psychiatric disease/diagnosis
Disorientation or fluctuating levels of consciousness
Presence of visual, tactile, or olfactory hallucinations

*Overlap is possible; exceptions to these exist.

Given that a history is often unobtainable in an intoxicated or violent patient, a thorough physical examination is important. One study showed that failure to perform an appropriate examination contributed to 43% of missed medical diagnoses in patients admitted from the ED to a psychiatric unit [6]. EPs should take precautions to ensure that this evaluation is done completely and safely. The patient's cervical spine should be immobilized if the possibility of trauma exists. A complete set of vital signs should be measured and reviewed on every patient, including the temperature. Fever in the presence of new psychiatric symptoms suggests an infectious etiology. Patients who abuse alcohol or certain stimulants are at particular risk for hypothermia and hyperthermia, respectively. A bedside glucose measurement should be considered the sixth "vital sign." Hypoglycemia is a readily correctable life-threatening cause of altered mental status in an apparently intoxicated or violent patient. Many chronic alcoholics have malnutrition and depleted glycogen stores, placing them at increased risk of hypoglycemia.

It is important that patients are disrobed prior to the physical examination. Although this is often met with protest by the patient and staff, EPs must aggressively search for clues to medical illnesses or occult trauma. Disrobing patients allows for weapon searches, which minimizes the possibility of self-inflicted or staff injuries. Keys and wallets left in back pockets may cause skin lacerations and neurapraxias; these items should be removed. Without their clothing, keys, wallets, or shoes, patients are less likely to leave the ED before their evaluation is completed.

The neurologic examination is particularly useful in correctly identifying medical conditions in both intoxicated and violent patients. Unfortunately, it is frequently neglected, incompletely or incorrectly performed, or not documented [1, 5]. In a random sample of 120 EPs from 1983, Zun found that few EPs performed an entire mental status examination (MSE); 72% took <5 min to perform one, using selected, unvalidated components [7]. In another study, failure to perform an adequate MSE was the single most important error contributing to the misdiagnosis of patients inappropriately admitted to psychiatric units from EDs. In this study, none of the 64 misdiagnosed cases had an adequate MSE documented [6] (See appendices on page 106).

Serial reevaluations (including repeated vital signs) are prudent for every ED patient, especially those who are intoxicated. Intoxicated patients are at risk for delayed presentations of bleeding or aspiration. Those involved in motor vehicle collisions are five times more likely to have traumatic injuries missed during their ED evaluation [8]. Patients with chronic alcohol use can develop hypoglycemia and/or withdrawal. Frequent reevaluation helps ensure that illnesses with latent phases, such as toxic alcohol poisoning, are not missed. Although there is a great deal of variability, the mental status of most uncomplicated intoxicated patients normalizes 3–5 hr from ED admission [9]. Further work-up is warranted if the mental status deteriorates or fails to improve, or if new signs or symptoms develop, such as pain, focal neurologic or abnormal vital signs, or abdominal guarding. A low threshold should exist for laboratory and radiologic testing of patients with new psychiatric symptoms, medical comorbidities, and advanced age [7, 10].

Pitfall | **Inappropriate use of blood alcohol levels during management and disposition**

Ordering a serum blood alcohol level (BAL) on every suspected intoxicated patient is unnecessary. Such an approach is time–consuming, costly, may be invasive, and rarely changes patient management. Being selective about when and how to measure a BAL is recommended to prevent errors and delays in patient care, as well as to reduce costs.

> KEY FACT | **Intoxicated patients with BALs <200–240 mg/dl and a Glasgow Coma Scale (GCS) of 13 or less should be evaluated for additional causes of altered mental status.**

One circumstance in which the BAL is important is when differentiating altered mental status secondary to alcohol from alternative or additional causes, such as head trauma, metabolic disturbances, seizures, psychosis, or multiple drug overdose [11]. A BAL may also be useful when the diagnosis is uncertain or an intoxicated patient's mental status does not clear over time. One study of 918 consecutive trauma patients concluded that a patient's GCS is not statistically affected by alcohol until the BAL is 200 mg/dl or higher [12].

Another study evaluating GCS scores in intoxicated assault patients found that in most patients, a BAL >240 mg/dl did not reduce one's GCS by more than 2–3 points [13]. These studies suggest that intoxicated patients with BALs <200–240 mg/dl and a GCS of 13 or less should be evaluated for additional causes of altered mental status. For example, a patient with a GCS of 12 and a BAL of 80 mg/dl should be further evaluated for an alternative diagnosis or diagnoses. On the other hand, if a patient's BAL is consistent with the degree of altered mental status, then supportive care with frequent reevaluations is appropriate.

The results of a traditional serum BAL may take 30–120 min, which, in some circumstances, may cause dangerous delays in patient care. Breath and saliva analyses allow correlation of a patient's alcohol level with their clinical condition within 5 min. This rapid turnaround allows EPs to be more efficient if changes to patient management are necessary. These alternative methods are less expensive, require minimal training, and are as accurate as serum analysis if properly performed [14–17].

> KEY FACT | The rate of elimination of alcohol follows zero-order kinetics: about 12 mg/dl/hr in non-drinkers, 15 mg/dl/hr in social drinkers, and 30 mg/dl/hr in chronic drinkers.

Once the patient's alcohol level is known, repeat levels are rarely needed. Because alcohol is rapidly absorbed in the stomach, the level should be near its maximum when a patient arrives at the ED. After this, the rate of elimination of alcohol follows zero-order kinetics: about 12 mg/dl/hr in non-drinkers, 15 mg/dl/hr in social drinkers, and 30 mg/dl/hr in chronic drinkers [11]. Furthermore, relying on a repeat alcohol level to determine whether a patient is ready for discharge is inappropriate. More important than an actual level is the patient's decisional capacity and ability for airway control. Chronic users can function with minimal mental or motor dysfunction at levels as high as 400 mg/dl. In fact, waiting for the BAL to decrease in these patients not only may take many hours, but can also result in symptoms of withdrawal. Conversely, a patient with a BAL legally deemed safe to drive may still have motor or decisional deficits due to a lack of tolerance or an occult medical condition. Finally, using BALs for legal purposes is state-dependent. Several states have mandatory reporting laws or require EPs to disclose a BAL at police request. However, other states may require police to obtain a court order before EPs can share patient information, including BAL results, without consent.

Pitfall | **Failure to protect the patient, staff, and third parties from harm**

The uncontrolled behavior of some patients can hinder their evaluation and subsequent diagnosis of a serious medical condition. Such behavior can also cause self-inflicted injuries, as well as injuries to ED staff or innocent third parties. The challenge for EPs is to ensure such patients receive a comprehensive evaluation while protecting themselves and others.

Numerous studies show that ED personnel are at high risk for assault by agitated patients. In a survey of 127 EDs at US teaching hospitals, 43% reported physical attacks against staff at least once a month. In the preceding 5 years, 80% had at least one staff member injured by a violent patient, 57% reported at least one threat of violence with a weapon, including two hostage incidents, and 7% reported fatal violent acts. Eighteen percent of these EDs surveyed reported weapon threats at least once a month [18].

Recognizing historical and physical predictors of impending violence may prevent such attacks (see Tables 13.2 and 13.3). The best predictor of a violent episode is a previous history of violence [19]. Patients brought in under arrest also represent a high-risk group. Those individuals restrained by police prior to ED arrival will likely need restraints in the ED [20]. Another risk factor for impending violence is a history of psychiatric illness. Organic disorders such as dementia, delirium, chemical intoxication with alcohol or stimulant drugs, and alcohol or chemical withdrawal also possess high potential for violent behavior. Certain physical clues can help identify potentially violent patients as well. Patients who are easily startled, use pressured speech, pace, clench their fists, invade other people's personal space, or make abrupt body motions are more likely to behave violently [21, 22]. Another extremely important predictor of impending violence is a patient who provokes anxiety or fear in the ED staff [19]. These patients should always be presumed dangerous.

Once a potentially violent patient has been identified, most laws dictate that the least restrictive intervention is

Table 13.2 Historical clues that predict violent behavior.

Prior history of violence
Patient arrival to ED in police custody or in restraints
Known history of psychiatric illness
History of substance abuse, including intoxication or withdrawal

Table 13.3 Clues that predict violent behavior.

Acute intoxication with (or withdrawal from) alcohol or other drugs, especially stimulants
Startles easily
Pressured speech
Frequent pacing in room
Repeated clenching of fists
Invasion of other people's personal space
Abrupt body motions
Physically imposing individual
Clinical signs of prior altercations, such as scars, fight injuries, or bruises

employed to control behavior. Thus, de-escalation strategies should be attempted first. Minimizing the time a patient is kept waiting decreases the potential for violence. He or she should be checked for weapons and placed in a quiet, private environment with minimal external stimuli. The room should be free of dangerous objects (needles, equipment cords, laceration trays, pill bottles, etc.). Staff should be aware that many objects have been used to cause injury, such as IV poles, bedpans, or water basins. It is also important to separate patients from potentially violent family members and friends. Two recent studies established that between 11% and 89% of assaults against ED staff came from the family or friends of an agitated patient [23, 24]. Items to increase patient comfort and gain trust should be provided, such as blankets and/or food. The proper positioning of security may serve to de-escalate potentially violent situations as well as provide protection. Although it may compromise confidentiality, EPs should leave a potentially violent patient's door open during the evaluation, and remain between the patient and the door at all times [25].

It is important for EPs to appear calm, convey a sense of control, and express appropriate concern for the patient. Empathic verbal interventions and collaborative approaches are recommended by emergency psychiatrists and highly desired by agitated patients, but are not frequently instituted by EPs [19, 22, 26, 27]. These include repeating phrases back to the patient to demonstrate understanding (without necessarily agreeing), sharing concern, and involving the patient in treatment decisions when possible. The patient must not feel rushed. Another staff member should sit and calmly talk with the patient if the EP is too busy [22]. Providers should avoid prolonged eye contact with the patient, crossing their arms, or keeping their arms behind their backs, as these actions may threaten the patient and worsen agitation [19]. Other dangerous actions include ignoring a violent patient, arguing with him, ordering him to calm down, threatening to call security, or underestimating the inherent risk of the situation [28].

If less restrictive methods fail to de-escalate the situation, the next step is a "show of force" (also called a "show of numbers"). Patients who are not psychotic will usually cooperate on seeing several security personnel. If a patient continues to be a danger to himself or others, and/or a life-threatening injury cannot be ruled out, the patient may need to be restrained. Restraint options include chemical, physical, or both. If the situation warrants, and it becomes necessary to temporarily seclude a patient, extreme caution should be exercised. In 1982, the US Supreme Court made an historical decision that has served as legal precedent for seclusion and restraint use by EPs. In *Youngberg v. Romeo*, it was held that reasons definitely exist to restrain patients "to protect them as well as others from violence." Furthermore, "courts must show deference to the judgment exercised by a qualified professional" [29]. Since then, courts have upheld cases requiring restraints and procedures, without patient consent, to diagnosis and treat mentally incapacitated patients in emergency situations [30, 31]. Strict adherence to national, state, and hospital guidelines must be maintained to prevent or minimize untoward outcomes. Using seclusion or restraints to punish patients or for staff convenience is prohibited by the Joint Commission on Accreditation of Healthcare Organizations (JCAHO), Medicare regulations, and most state laws.

Pitfall | **Failure to consider the indications for and adverse effects of chemical restraint**

Many chemical restraints have similar efficacy and speed of onset for reducing acute agitation, but differ greatly in terms of specific indications, available formulations, adverse effects, cost, and patient preference. Medical outcomes and patient satisfaction can improve if these factors are considered prior to using chemical restraint.

Agitation from alcohol and benzodiazepine withdrawal, as well as cocaine and amphetamine hyperactivity, should be treated with benzodiazepines. Lorazepam (Ativan) is the only benzodiazepine absorbed well orally (PO), sublingually (SL), intramuscularly (IM), and intravenously (IV), and has no active metabolites. The typical dose for each route is 0.5–2 mg. Midazolam (Versed) may have a more rapid onset of action and a shorter duration of action than lorazepam. An effective starting dose of midazolam appears to be 5 mg IM [10]. Regardless of the benzodiazepine chosen, lower doses or alternative agents should be used in patients with alcohol intoxication, underlying chronic obstructive pulmonary disease (COPD), or the elderly to avoid excessive sedation, respiratory depression, and hypotension [32].

> KEY FACT | **A potential complication of most typical antipsychotics is QT-interval prolongation, which predisposes to ventricular dysrhythmias.**

Agitation from alcohol intoxication or known psychiatric illness can be effectively treated with haloperidol (Haldol), a high-potency butyrophenone or typical antipsychotic. The standard dose for younger patients is 5–10 mg PO/IM/IV. This dose is best reduced to 2 mg in the elderly or those with comorbidities. There is no risk of respiratory depression or hypotension, but distressing extrapyramidal symptoms can occur. These can be avoided or treated with doses of 2 mg benztropine (Cogentin), 25–50 mg diphenhydramine (Benadryl), or 2 mg lorazepam PO/IM/IV. Akathisia (the sensation of uneasiness and motor restlessness) should not be confused with worsening agitation, and should not be treated with repeat doses of antipsychotics. Another potential complication of most typical antipsychotics is QT-interval prolongation, which predisposes to ventricular dysrhythmias. Patients at greatest risk appear to have cardiac problems, electrolyte disturbances, or take medications with quinidine-like cardiac effects. The high potency butyrophenone droperidol (Inapsine), a favorite of many EPs for acute agitation, was recently taken off the market in Europe and given a Black Box warning in the US due to concerns about QT-interval prolongation leading to dysrhythmias. Many authors have disputed these findings, and, despite these concerns, prefer droperidol 5 mg IM/IV for more rapid sedation compared to haloperidol [10, 26, 32].

In 2006, the American College of Emergency Physicians (ACEP) issued a clinical policy statement giving a level B recommendation for the use of benzodiazepines (lorazepam or midazolam) or typical antipsychotics (haloperidol or droperidol) as monotherapy for undifferentiated causes of acute agitation [10]. The combination of a benzodiazepine and an antipsychotic is felt to cause fewer extrapyramidal symptoms, and allows less of each drug to be used [26, 32]. One popular regimen for emergency control of acute agitation is 5 mg haloperidol and 2 mg lorazepam IM.

The use of atypical antipsychotics has recently been replacing the use of typical antipsychotics in the outpatient setting, including psychiatric EDs. The atypical antipsychotics appear to be as effective as the typical antipsychotics, with less risk of extrapyramidal side effects. There also appears to be an overall decreased incidence of QT prolongation. In its clinical policy, ACEP gives a level B recommendation for the use of these agents as monotherapy for acutely agitated patients with known psychiatric illness [10]. Risperidone (Risperdal) is available as a liquid as well as an oral disintegrating tablet (ODT), which can be useful for cooperative patients who are moderately agitated. The typical dose is 2 mg PO. However, risperidone's utility is limited in severely combative and uncooperative patients because there currently is no rapidly-acting IM preparation. Olanzapine (Zyprexa) can be used as an ODT for moderately agitated patients or IM for severely agitated patients. A dose of 10 mg IM appears to be safe and effective for most patients, with half that dose for the elderly or debilitated. Because of possible risks of bradycardia and hypotension, olanzapine should not be given within 1 hr of a benzodiazepine. Therefore, it should be used with extreme caution in patients with alcohol or sedative intoxication. Ziprasidone (Geodon) is a new agent for severely agitated or uncooperative patients. The most effective dose appears to be 20 mg IM. There is concern over measurable prolongation of the QT interval, although these findings have been refuted by some studies [26, 32, 33]. Research is ongoing to identify the safest and most effective pharmacologic agent or combination of agents for controlling all causes of acute agitation.

Consumer groups and consensus guidelines from emergency psychiatrists recommend that patients be asked to willingly take medications whenever possible prior to administering them by force, as this increases patient satisfaction and improves therapeutic alliance. It is also recommended to ask patients about a history of response to or adverse effects from chemical restraints prior to selecting a particular medication. Most patients prefer benzodiazepines to decrease acute agitation, followed by atypical antipsychotics. Patients least prefer conventional antipsychotics. Not surprisingly, patients overwhelmingly prefer the oral administration of any drug to involuntary IM administration [26, 27].

Regardless of the medication(s) chosen, it is important to be aware that the half-life of some of these agents is several hours. For patients who are being released (ideally to the care of responsible adults) or transferred to psychiatric facilities, potential side effects of these medications must be anticipated and communicated.

Pitfall | **Incomplete or dangerous physical restraint application**

Physical restraints are often necessary in addition to chemical restraints. On rare occasions, physical restraints may be used instead of chemical restraints. However, their use can be dangerous not only from a medical perspective, but also from a legal one. Because of their inherent risks, any use of physical restraints requires proper technique, frequent reevaluation, and meticulous documentation.

Many healthcare workers have been injured during attempts to restrain combative patients. To reduce the likelihood of injury, no one should restrain a patient alone. Ideally, a six-person team should do this – one for each extremity, one to control the head, and one leader to apply the restraints. Every team member should have pre-assigned roles, having received education in and previously rehearsed restraint application. Team members should remove objects that could be used as weapons against them, such as stethoscopes, eyeglasses, neckties or scarves, pens, scissors, or lapel pins. Similar to a well-run cardiac resuscitation, only the team leader should give orders. The team should advance to the patient from all directions on the leader's command. Prior to their application, the patient should have the reason for restraints explained. There should be no negotiation once the decision to restrain has been made.

Patient-related complications from physical restraints are probably under-reported in the literature. Lavoie's survey showed that in the preceding 5 years, 13% of EDs had caused significant patient injuries from restraints; 16% were sued over restraining a patient, failing to restrain a patient, or injuries sustained by a patient during restraint application or while restrained [18]. Restraints must be secure enough to prevent injury or escape, but loose enough to prevent neurovascular complications. Leather restraints applied to both ankles and wrists are the safest and most secure [21, 22, 26]. One common error made by ED staff is incompletely restraining a patient, which allows the patient to harm himself, others, or release his or her restraints and elope. Patients can remove restraints applied only to the legs or only to one arm. Cloth or soft restraints should not be used because they are less secure than leather restraints. Gauze bandages are discouraged because they risk neurovascular injury to the extremities. Other protective measures include soft cervical collars to prevent head banging. A nonrebreather oxygen mask connected to high flow oxygen can protect staff from spitting, as can placing a clear shield over the patient's face. Once restraints are applied, they should remain in place only as long as the reason for their use remains.

> KEY FACT | **Restraints must be applied in the least restrictive manner possible for the shortest period of time.**

It is equally important that restraints are applied properly to prevent iatrogenic injuries. Skin tears, fractures, dislocations, and head injuries have been reported, as has dehydration. In the past 10 years, over 130 deaths have been reported from restraints in all settings [34]. The number one cause of these deaths is inadequate staff orientation to and training in the use of restraints [35]. One ED active in research in this area reviewed its own restraint-related complications. It identified documented complications only 7% of the time during the year analyzed. Severe injuries and deaths related to restraints were not reported [36]. A 2004 survey found that a large percentage of EM residencies and pediatric EM fellowships do not teach the proper application of physical restraints or the appropriate situations in which restraints should be used [37]. These findings suggest that hospitals and training programs should increase formal education on, including simulated exposure to, restraining patients.

The most common cause of restraint-related death is asphyxiation [38]. Patients restrained in the prone position, including those brought to the ED by police in hobble restraints ("hog-tied") may be at greatest risk. The prone position can cause airway obstruction and restriction of the diaphragm and intercostal muscles. When prone-restrained agitated patients struggle with police or ED staff, catecholamine surges can quickly result in unmet oxygen demands. Hypoxia, cardiac dysrhythmias, and sudden death may ensue [38, 39]. Other actions which cause asphyxia include putting a sheet over the patient's head, "burying" the patient's head into the gurney, and inadvertently obstructing the patient's airway when pulling his arms across his neck [40].

Deaths while restrained have also been reported by strangulation. Patients with waist or vest restraints have strangled themselves when trying to get out of confinement. Patients who are altered and/or combative are also at high risk for entrapment of the head, neck, or thorax in the spaces created by side rails. To prevent this, patients should be securely restrained to gurney rails; gaps no greater than 5 in. should be present between the mattress and the side rails.

In response to restraint-related complications in various settings, the Centers for Medicare and Medicaid Services (CMS) and JCAHO implemented regulations concerning the proper use of restraints. Only physicians or other licensed independent practitioners (LIPs) can order restraints, which must be done in the least restrictive manner possible for the least specified period of time. If an adult patient is placed in restraints by other staff members, a physician or LIP must evaluate the patient within 1 hr [42, 43]. Once restrained, patients must be continually monitored. This is important because the second most common cause of restraint-related deaths is inadequate patient assessment [35]. Besides assessing for complications, patients must be evaluated for underlying illnesses. One ED study reported that nearly 50% of patients restrained for behavioral reasons ultimately required medical or surgical admissions [44].

Finally, documentation should be complete when using chemical or physical restraints, or both. Meticulous documentation is the best defense against potential future investigations of battery and false imprisonment lawsuits. The medical record should document the following:

1. The emergent indication for restraint (i.e., the patient was a danger to himself or others, and a comprehensive evaluation was impossible without restraints).
2. The need for restraints and treatment was explained to the patient. If the patient lacked the mental capacity to understand the nature of his condition and the risks/benefits of treatment versus no treatment, this must be documented.
3. Less restrictive options had been tried and failed.
4. The type of restraints used, and that no injuries were sustained during their application (or any injuries that occurred).
5. Orders for and the results of frequent reassessments, position changes, and vital signs [21].

Pitfall | **Failure to assess for and recognize suicide and/or homicide risk**

> KEY FACT | **Alcohol intoxication increases suicide risk. 40–60% of people who commit suicide are intoxicated with alcohol at the time of their death.**

Many EPs ignore the suicidal statements of intoxicated patients, assuming they are "just drunk" or "don't really mean it." These are dangerous assumptions given that 40–60% of people who commit suicide are intoxicated with alcohol at the time of their death [45]. Alcohol intoxication increases suicide risk in both chronic and occasional drinkers [46]. It impairs judgment, increases aggressiveness and impulsiveness, and may potentiate or obscure the presence of dangerous co-ingestants. Patients who are alcohol-dependent also often have additional independent risk factors for suicide, such as psychiatric illness or social and financial problems [45].

Patients who express suicidal ideations should be carefully observed and restrained if necessary. Once patients are no longer intoxicated, it is important to ascertain their suicidal intent prior to their release. A low threshold to consult a psychiatrist or psychologist trained in evaluating suicidal risk should exist. Releasing intoxicated patients once they are sober without reassessment or intervention affords patients who are suicidal "only when intoxicated" the opportunity to consider or attempt suicide the next time they become intoxicated [47].

Suicide and homicide are closely linked. People who threaten homicide are more likely to commit suicide. It is therefore important to screen violent patients for both homicidal and suicidal ideations prior to disposition. Similarly, staff must be aware of the potential for violence in suicidal patients [47]. Any patient who is a threat to himself or others can be involuntarily committed for a finite period of time. In addition, if a specific threat of violence is made against an identifiable third party, many jurisdictions have ruled that physicians have the duty to break physician–patient confidentially and warn law enforcement agencies and potential victim(s) [48–50].

Pitfall | **Failure to provide brief interventions and appropriate substance abuse referrals to intoxicated patients**

In the US, approximately 7.6 million ED visits annually are alcohol related, representing 7.9% of total ED visits [51]. Between 20% and 30% of the patients seen in US hospital EDs have underlying alcohol problems; as high as 38% are legally intoxicated [52, 53]. This large prevalence of alcohol problems costs the US $185 billion annually, with 20% of the total national expenditure for hospital care related to alcohol [53, 54]. These statistics are alarming given that alcohol-related injuries and illnesses are preventable.

Many EPs underestimate the importance of providing brief interventions to ED patients, despite numerous studies demonstrating the effectiveness that such interventions have at decreasing future alcohol consumption [54–62]. A review of at least 12 randomized trials and 32 controlled studies in 14 countries concluded that brief interventions are more effective than no counseling, and, in many patients, as effective as more extensive treatment [63]. As little as 5 min of advice has been shown to be valuable to patients [60]. Interventions should focus on empathetically providing feedback about the drinking, stressing patient responsibility and control, and negotiating a strategy for change [64]. Conducting interventions in the ED capitalizes on the crucial *teachable moment*; patients are most motivated to change when suffering from the consequences of their drinking. In addition, brief interventions require minimal training and can be performed by a variety of people: doctors, nurses, social workers, care coordinators, staff members, and even community workers [55, 59].

The benefits of screening patients and conducting brief interventions are enormous. A 2005 cost–benefit analysis of intoxicated accident victims demonstrated that the net cost savings of one intervention was $330 for each patient. The benefit in reduced health care expenditures was a savings of $3.81 for every $1.00 spent on screening and intervention. If interventions were routinely offered to eligible injured adult patients nationwide, the potential net savings could approach $1.82 billion annually [65].

Because of these potential benefits, *Healthy People 2010* (the disease prevention agenda for the US) has listed among its goals for this decade to increase the proportion of patients referred for follow-up care of alcohol or drug problems after diagnosis or treatment in hospital EDs [66]. To achieve this objective, the Society for Academic Emergency Medicine (SAEM) Substance Abuse Task Force recommends that every ED establish a referral system for substance abusers. Phone numbers and directions to local resources, such as detoxification centers, community outpatient treatment programs, family counseling, Alcoholics Anonymous (AA) meetings, and AA sponsors should be available and provided to those in need [64].

Pitfall | **Prematurely releasing an intoxicated or violent patient**

The decision to discharge an intoxicated or violent patient from the ED must be made carefully. Extended liability laws can hold a physician responsible if a patient is released and consequently injures himself or a third party. Unfortunately, the premature release of intoxicated or violent patients is a common pitfall. Often, their loud and disruptive demands for discharge are enthusiastically and hastily met. Sometimes, a patient's demands for premature discharge IS misguidedly justified by having HIM sign out against medical advice (AMA). Whatever the reason, it is crucial that patient safety and the safety of third parties, as well as any legal requirements, are considered prior to release. The most important element in the decision to comply with a patient's demands for premature discharge is his decision-making capacity. The patient must be able to understand and compare the risks and benefits of various options. The patient's choice should remain consistent over time and be clearly communicated [67]. Adults who are neither suicidal nor homicidal and have full decisional capacity can refuse treatment, be discharged, or leave AMA if they have been fully informed about and comprehend the risks and alternatives to their decision. If a patient's mental status prevents him from having the necessary decision-making capacity, he cannot be discharged alone or sign out AMA. Such a patient must be detained in the ED until his mental status has improved. Alternatively, it may be appropriate in certain situations to release a patient to the care of a responsible adult who can drive safely and return or call 911 if problems develop. It is important to remember that alcohol consumption or an elevated BAL does not necessarily mean that a patient lacks decisional capacity.

It is not permissible to use a psychiatric hold in order to detain an intoxicated or aggressive patient unless very clear conditions are met (danger to self, danger to others, or gravely disabled). However, many EDs have what is commonly referred to as an "ED Hold," in which ED policy at that institution allows security to prevent a patient from leaving. Another alternative is contacting the police, who can encourage patients to listen to instructions or behave in a more appropriate manner. It is advisable to have clear guidelines and be familiar with institutional policies, as these situations occur commonly.

> KEY FACT | **Any patient who is released AMA should have documentation of full decisional capacity, and that he has been fully informed about the risks and benefits of all options.**

Appropriate documentation is crucial. Documentation of a final reassessment, including vital signs, and a lack of suicidal or homicidal ideations should occur, with the date and time. Any patient who is released AMA should have documentation of full decisional capacity, and that he has been fully informed about the risks and benefits of all options. For an intoxicated patient, outpatient referrals should be provided, and the patient should be instructed not to drink and drive. These instructions should be documented as well. If possible, document that the patient was discharged to the care of a responsible adult driver to whom the discharge instructions were provided, explained, and understood. For a patient who elopes from the ED, efforts used to prevent elopement, attempts to find or contact the patient, and notification of the appropriate authorities and third parties should be documented.

Pearls for Improving Patient Outcomes

- A comprehensive medical evaluation is essential to rule out alternative or co-existing medical conditions resulting in or from an intoxicated or violent state.
- There are a few specific circumstances when a BAL is necessary; consider using rapid saliva or breath tests if these are available.
- Predictors of violent behavior should be recognized. Necessary measures to protect the patient, staff, and third parties, such as de-escalation techniques, seclusion, and restraints should be used.
- Chemical restraints should be administered based on suspected diagnosis and known adverse effects. Whenever possible, involve the patient in the selection of the medication and ask him/her to take it willingly.
- Physical restraint application should be rehearsed. Restraints should be applied to each extremity completely, safely, and with frequent reevaluation.

- The potential for suicide and homicide in intoxicated or violent patients must not be overlooked or minimized.
- The ED is a cost-effective and ideal place for providing brief interventions and social services to individuals who abuse alcohol or other substances.
- Do not allow patients who lack decision-making capacity to elope or be discharged AMA.
- Appropriate documentation is essential. Mental status examinations, frequent reevaluations, reasons for restraints, lack of suicidality or homicidality, notification of appropriate authorities and potential victims, and social service referrals should be clearly documented.

Appendix A

Mini-Mental State (MMS) examination, from Folstein MF, Folstein SE, McHugh PR. " Mini-Mental State:" A Practical Method for Grading the Cognitive State of Patients for the Clinician. *J. Psych. Res.* 1975; 12(3)189–198.

Appendix B

Confusion Assessment Method, from Inouye SK, van Dyck CH, Alessi CA, et al. Clarifying Confusion. The Confusion Assessment Method. *Ann Intern Med* 1990; 113:941–948.

References

1. Tintinalli JE, Peacock FW, Wright MA. Emergency medical evaluation of psychiatric patients. *Ann Emerg Med* 1994; 23(4): 859–62.
2. Hall R, Gardner E, Stickney S, et al. Physical illness manifesting as psychiatric disease. II. Analysis of a state hospital inpatient population. *Arch Gen Psych* 1980; 37(9):989–995.
3. Henneman PL, Mendoza R, Lewis RS. Prospective evaluation of emergency department medical clearance. *Ann Emerg Med* 1994; 24(4):672–7.
4. Dubin WR, Weiss KJ, Zeccardi JA. Organic brain syndrome. The psychiatric imposter. *J Am Med Assoc* 1983; 249(1):60–2.
5. Lagomasino I, Daly R, Stoudemire A. Medical assessment of patients presenting with psychiatric symptoms in the emergency setting. *Psych Clin N Am* 1999; 22(4):819–50.
6. Reeves RR, Pendarvis EJ, Kimble R. Unrecognized medical emergencies admitted to psychiatric units. *Am J Emerg Med* 2000; 18(4):390–3.
7. Zun LS. Evidence-based evaluation of psychiatric patients. *J Emerg Med* 2005; 28(1):35–9.
8. Fabrri A, Marchesini G, Morselli-Labate A, et al. Blood alcohol concentration and management of road trauma patients in the emergency department. *J Trauma* 2001; 50(3):521–8.
9. Todd K, Berk WA, Welch RD, et al. Prospective analysis of mental status progression in ethanol-intoxicated patients. *Am J Emerg Med* 1992; 10(4):271–3.
10. Lukens TW, Wolf SJ, Edlow JA, et al. American College of Emergency Physicians Clinical Policies Subcommittee (Writing Committee) on critical issues in the diagnosis and management

of the adult psychiatric patient in the emergency department. *Ann Emerg Med* 2006; 47(1):79–99.

11. Gibb K. Serum alcohol levels, toxicology screens, and use of the breath alcohol analyzer. *Ann Emerg Med* 1986; 15(3):349–53.

12. Galbraith S, Murray W, Patel A, et al. The relationship between alcohol and head injury and its effect on the conscious level. *Br J Surg* 1976; 63(2):128–30.

13. Brickley M, Shepherd J. The relationship between alcohol intoxication, injury severity and Glasgow Coma Score in assault patients. *Injury* 1995; 26(5):311–14.

14. Keim ME, Bartfield JM, Raccio-Robak N. Blood ethanol estimation: a comparison of three methods. *Acad Emerg Med* 1996; 3(1):85–7.

15. Smolle K, Hofmann G, Kaufmann P, et al. QED alcohol test: a simple and quick method to detect ethanol in saliva of patients in emergency departments. Comparison with the conventional determination in blood. *Intens Care Med* 1999; 25(5): 492–5.

16. Degutis L, Rabinovici R, Sabbaj A, et al. The saliva strip test is an accurate method to determine blood alcohol concentration in trauma patients. *Acad Emerg Med* 2004; 11(8):885–7.

17. Gibb K, Oak R, Yee A, et al. Accuracy and usefulness of a breath alcohol analyzer. *Ann Emerg Med* 1984; 13(7):516–20.

18. Lavoie FW, Carter G, Danzi D, et al. Emergency department violence in United States teaching hospitals. *Ann Emerg Med* 1998; 17(11):1227–33.

19. Hill S, Petit J. The violent patient. *Emerg Med Clin N Am* 2000; 18(2):301–15.

20. Blomhoff S, Seim S, Friis S. Can prediction of violence among psychiatric inpatients be improved? *Hosp Comm Psychiatr* 1990; 41(7):771–5.

21. Salkin M. Use of restraints and seclusion in the ED. *ED Legal Letter* 1998; 9(6):57–68.

22. Dubin W. Violent patients. In: Bosker, G. (ed.), *The Emergency Medicine Reports Textbook of Adult and Pediatric Emergency Medicine.* 2nd edition. Atlanta, Georgia: American Health Consultants Incorporated, 2002, pp. 2069–76.

23. Kowalenko T, Walters BL, Khare RK, et al. Workplace violence: a survey of emergency physicians in the state of Michigan. *Ann Emerg Med* 2005; 46(2):142–7.

24. Ayranci U. Violence toward health care workers in emergency departments in west Turkey. *J Emerg Med* 2005; 28(3): 361–5.

25. Meyers T, Garmel GM. Abnormal behavior. In: Mahadevan SV, Garmel GM (eds), *An Introduction to Clinical Emergency Medicine: Guide for Practitioners in the Emergency Department.* Cambridge, UK: Cambridge University Press, 2005, pp. 161–70.

26. Allen MH, Currier GW, Hughes DH, et al. Treatment of behavioral emergencies. *Post Grad Med* May 2001: 1–88.

27. Allen M, Carpenter D, Sheets J, et al. What do consumers say they want and need during a psychiatric emergency? *J Psych Practice* 2003; 9(1):39–58.

28. Rice M, Moore G. Management of the violent patient. Therapeutic and legal considerations. *Emerg Med Clinics of N Am* 1991; 9(1):13–30.

29. *Youngberg v. Romeo*, 457 US 307 (1982).

30. *Miller v. Rhode Island Hospital*, 625 A.2d 778, 785 (R.I. 1993).

31. *Blackman v. Rifkin*, 759 P.2d 54, 58 (Colo Ct. App 1988).

32. Battaglia J. Pharmacological management of acute agitation. *Drugs* 2005; 65(9):1207–22.

33. Zimbroff DL, Allen MH, Battaglia J. Best clinical practice with ziprasidone IM: update after 2 years of experience. *CNS Spectrums* 2005; 10(9):1–15.

34. Joint Commission for Accreditation of Healthcare Organizations. *Sentinel Event Statistics.* September 30, 2005, www.jcaho.org

35. Joint Commission for Accreditation of Healthcare Organizations. *Root Causes of Restraint Deaths (1995–2004).* May 13, 2002, www.jcaho.org

36. Zun LS. A prospective study of the complication rate of use of patient restraint in the emergency department. *J Emerg Med* 2003; 24(2):119–24.

37. Dorfman DH, Kastner B. The use of restraint for pediatric psychiatric patients in emergency departments. *Pediatr Emerg Care* 2004; 20(3):151–6.

38. Mohr WK, Petti TA, Mohr BD. Adverse effects associated with physical restraint. *Can J Psych* 2003; 48(5):330–7.

39. Abdon-Beckman D. An awkward position: restraints and sudden death. *J Emerg Med Ser* 1997; 22(3):88–94.

40. Joint Commission for Accreditation of Healthcare Organizations. *Sentinel Event Alert: Preventing Restraint Deaths.* Issue 8, November 18, 1998. www.jcaho.org

41. FDA Safety Alert: Entrapment Hazards with Hospital Bed Side Rails, 1995.

42. Joint Commission for Accreditation of Healthcare Organizations. PC.12.130 and PC.12.140. Revised April 1, 2005. www.jcaho.org

43. Centers for Medicare & Medicaid Services. *Conditions of Participation for Hospitals.* 482.13. Revised October 1, 1999. www.cms.hhs.gov

44. Lavoie FW. Consent, involuntary treatment, and the use of force in an urban emergency department. *Ann Emerg Med* 1992; 21(1):25–32.

45. Mental health and suicide facts. Department of Health and Human Services. National Strategy for Suicide Prevention; 2004. http://www.mentalhealth.org/suicideprevention/suicidefacts.asp

46. Hufford MR. Alcohol and suicide behavior. *Clin Psych Rev* 2001; 21(5):797–811.

47. Dwyer B. The suicidal patient. In: Bosker, G. (ed.), *The Emergency Medicine Reports Textbook of Adult and Pediatric Emergency Medicine.* 2nd edition. Atlanta, Georgia: American Health Consultants Incorporated, 2002, pp. 2053–60.

48. *Tarasoff v. Regents of the University of California*, 17 Cal. 3d 425, 131 Cal. Rptr. 14, 551 P.2d 334 (1976).

49. *Thompson v. County of Alameda*, 27 Cal. 3d 741, 167 Cal. Rptr. 70, 614 P.2d 728 (1980).

50. *Brady v. Hopper*, 570 F. Supp. 1333, 1338 D. Colo. 1983.

51. McDonald A, Wang N, Camargo C. US emergency department visits for alcohol-related diseases and injuries between 1992 and 2000. *Arch Intern Med* 2004; 164(5):531–7.

52. Centers for Disease Control and Prevention. *Injury Fact Book.* 2002. www.cdc.gov/ncipc/fact_book/09_Alcohol_%20Injuries_%20ED.htm

53. D'Onofrio G, Bernstein E, Bernstein J, et al. Patients with alcohol problems in the emergency department, Part 1: Improving detection. SAEM Substance Abuse Task Force. *Acad Emerg Med* 1998; 5(12):1200–9.

54. D'Onofrio G, Degutis LC. Preventive care in the emergency department: screening and brief intervention for alcohol problems in the emergency department: a systematic review. *Acad Emerg Med* 2002; 9(6):627–38.

55. Bernstein E, Bernstein J, Levenson S. Project ASSERT: an ED-based intervention to increase access to primary care, preventive services, and the substance abuse treatment system. *Ann Emerg Med* 1997; 30(2):181–9.

56. Wright LM, Moran L, Meyrick M, et al. Intervention by an alcohol health worker in an accident and emergency department. *Alcohol* 1998; 33:651–6.

57. Crawford M, Patton R, Touquet R, et al. Screening and referral for brief intervention of alcohol-misusing patients in an emergency department: a pragmatic randomized controlled trial. *Lancet* 2004; 364(9442):1334–9.

58. Green M, Setchell J, Hames P, et al. Management of alcohol abusing patients in accident and emergency departments. *J R Soc Med* 1993; 86(7):393–5.

59. Gentilello LM, Rivara FP, Donovan DM, et al. Alcohol interventions in a trauma center as a means of reducing the risk of injury recurrence. *Ann Surg* 1999; 230(4):473–80.

60. Babor TF, Acuda W, Campillo C, et al. World Health Organization Brief Intervention Study Group. A cross-national trial of brief intervention with heavy drinkers. *Am J Public Health* 1996; 86:948–55.

61. Wilk A, Jensen N, Havighurst T. Meta-analysis of randomized control trials addressing brief interventions in heavy alcohol drinkers. *J Gen Intern Med* 1997; 12(5):274–83.

62. Monti PM, Colby SM, Barnett NP, et al. Brief intervention for harm reduction with alcohol-positive older adolescents in a hospital emergency department. *J Consult Clin Psych* 1999; 67(6):989–94.

63. Bien TH, Miller WR, Tonigan JS. Brief interventions for alcohol problems: a review. *Addiction* 1993; 88(3):315–35.

64. D'Onofrio G, Bernstein E, Bernstein J, et al. Patients with alcohol problems in the emergency department, Part 2: Intervention and referral. *Acad Emerg Med* 1998; 5(12):1210–17.

65. Gentilello LM, Ebel B, Wickizer T, et al. Alcohol interventions for trauma patients treated in emergency departments and hospitals: a cost benefit analysis. *Ann Surg* 2005; 241(4):541–50.

66. US Department of Health and Human Services. *Healthy People 2010: Understanding and Improving Health*. Washington, DC: US Government Printing Office, 2000.

67. Marco C, Derse A. Leaving against medical advice: should you take no for an answer? *ED Legal Letter* 2004; 15(11):121–32.

Index